Alcoholism

Causes, Symptoms, Effects and Treatment

Alcoholism
Causes, Symptoms, Effects and Treatment

Edited by

Dr. Vinod K. Shanwal
Head, Dept. of Education and Training
School of Humanities and Social Sciences
Gautam Buddha University, Greater Noida

★★★

Dr. B.S. Chhikara
Department of Chemistry
Aditi Mahavidyalaya, University of Delhi

Manakin
PRESS

First published 2022
by CRC Press
4 Park Square, Milton Park, Abingdon, Oxon, OX14 4RN

and by CRC Press
6000 Broken Sound Parkway NW, Suite 300, Boca Raton, FL 33487-2742

CRC Press is an imprint of Informa UK Limited

British Library Cataloguing-in-Publication Data
A catalogue record for this book is available from the British Library

Library of Congress Cataloging-in-Publication Data
A catalog record has been requested

ISBN: 978-1-032-24840-0 (hbk)
ISBN: 978-1-003-28036-1 (ebk)

DOI: 10.1201/9781003280361

Manakin PRESS

Contents

Foreword

It is estimated that 4% of all the world's health problems are linked to excessive alcohol consumption. This form of alcohol use is a major health risk factor which eventually leads to chronic disability and possible death. Emphasis should be placed on effective strategies to help people who are dependent on alcohol. This would help to reduce excessive drinking, maintain sobriety, and prevent relapse.

Clinical studies have shown that approximately 8% of hospitalized patients suffer from complications related to alcohol withdrawal. Symptoms present as life- threatening condition that usually affects people when they try to decrease or discontinue their alcohol intake.

There have been advancements made in the health sciences for the improved treatment and rehabilitation of those who are either addicted to alcohol or are casual drinkers that have decided to quit. The awareness in certain sections of society has facilitated the formulation of policies or legal measures relating to the control of the sale and consumption of these substances.

Health care research has shown that a high number of motor vehicle accidents occur due to the easy availability of alcohol on the main highways. On 15th December 2016, The Honorable Supreme Court of India decided that all liquor shops and bars must be moved away from major highways.

During our present time, it is important to aggressively educate people on the harmful effects of alcohol consumption, involve family members, and bring in more stringent laws to control this debilitating predicament. Different stakeholders should come together and suggest ideas to prevent, reduce, control, or rehabilitate such persons.

This book has presented a very thorough and holistic view of current alcohol related issues. It includes chapters on social, economic, medical, and rehabilitation strategies. I believe that individuals, researchers, administrators, educators, health care policy planners, and medical professionals will gain insight from the information presented in this book.

Dr. Jaspreet S. Bains, MD
Department of Psychiatry
University of Pittsburgh Medical Center
(UPMC Altoona), Pennsylvania, U.S.A.

Foreword

Use of alcohol has existed in the society since the ancient period. Adverse effects of alcohol use have been identified since last many decades and are debated by health professionals, sociologists, economists, administrators, and psychologists. In the last few decades, use of alcohol in the society has increased a lot despite increasing awareness about its ill effects on health, and alcohol being a recognised cause in a number of accidents. Alcohol consumption is rampant in certain parts of our country, while some states have taken the route of legislation to ban it or reduce the harm of its effects. Role of social workers, opinion makers, health planners, researchers, health professionals and law reinforcement agencies is very crucial to reduce the harms associated with alcohol

Persons consuming alcohol are at a higher risk of developing diseases due to its direct toxic effects on different body systems, or indirectly through its effects on one's judgment leading to distorted functioning and accidents. Almost every anatomical and physiological system is adversely affected by the consumption of alcohol. Use of alcohol is also associated with nutritional deficiencies, leading to its own adverse consequences. The gastro-intestinal system (including liver and kidneys), central nervous system and cardio-vascular system are affected directly, as alcohol has direct toxic effects on these system. Use of alcohol is also associated with impaired decision making, cognitive deterioration, absenteeism, unemployment, a range of psychiatric disorders including depression, adjustment disorders, amnesic disorder, Wenicke encephalopathy, and dementia, and also increased risk of suicide. It is also a common cause of domestic violence, marital discord and many road traffic and industrial accidents.

There is a need to create awareness about the ill effects of alcohol in the society and motivating the alcohol users to stop it. Persons who want to leave it should be offered all kinds of help and easy access to services offering such help

The book "Alcoholism Causes, Symptoms, Effects and Treatment" edited by VK Shanwal and BS Chhikara gives a multidimensional view about alcoholism, as seen by professionals from a range of disciplines The book covers topics like factors leading to alcohol use disorders, its adverse effects, prohibition policy, its association with crime and how a person with alcohol problem can be helped. I commend the editors as well as the authors for their herculean effort and hope that this book serves as an excellent resource material for the persons interested in knowing causation, and adverse social and health effects of alcohol.

Dr. Rakesh K Chadda
Professor & Head
Department of Psychiatry and
Chief, National Drug Dependence Treatment Centre
All India Institute of Medical Sciences
New Delhi 110029

Preface

Alcoholism leads to physical, mental, psychological and social degradation of an individual. An alcoholic person is not only an economic burden on the family but also a source of continuous psychological strain which leads to disruption in mutual relationships with family and friends. Remedy to such a problem lies in combining together psychotherapies, medical care and de-addiction efforts of family and friends. Research on multi-dimensional aspects of alcoholism problems is intended in the chapters for a comprehensive solution to the problem. The chapters cover a wide range of topics on the theme of Alcoholism starting from health risks involved to the remedial measures available in medical as well as psychological fields.

Alcoholism may have many causes and people with certain personalities are more prone to it. Factors such as genetics, childhood influences, antisocial behavior, and personality traits also contribute towards menace of alcoholism in individuals. Personality traits like extroversion, neuroticism, conscientiousness, agreeableness and openness to experience influence the addiction in individuals. Cultural values and beliefs, and childhood experiences to govern thought process are indirectly related to earlier stages of alcohol addiction. Family history and life stress have implications on individual/s susceptibility to alcohol addiction.

Alcoholism not only affects the health of the addicted person but also relationship with the family members. Chronic intake of alcohol may have varied impact on the parenting, marital relationship, social image, communication and cohesion. The family may react to alcoholism differently depending upon the stage/phase of the drinking behavior; subsequently resulting in disruption of normal family routine and functions. Family cohesion also has a role to play in the diverse response towards the addicted person, greater cohesion within the family helps in prevention of addiction problems. Non-cohesion and over-cohesion both result in addiction cases. Similarly, communication within a family is also important in dealing with the addicted person.

The effects of alcoholism on the brain, is a study of the adverse effects of ethanol or "ethyl alcohol" on brain functioning and development. The sedative and depressant effects of ethanol results in the damaging of CNS and also may lead to malfunctioning of other vital organs. Alcohol influences neurotransmitter system in the brain, memory of the addicted person, behavior etc. Although the amount of damage depend on a variety of factors like age, gender, quantity of consumption and drinking pattern, alcoholism is a serious health risk not only for the brain but also for liver, respiratory system and psychological condition of the individual.

The Nutritional Deficiencies associated with Alcoholism explores the consequences of alcoholism that may lead to nutritional deficiencies and subsequently diseases. Lack of vitamins A,D,C,E and K lead to diseases like night blindness, softening of bones, delayed blood clotting thereby posing serious health risks for individuals addicted to alcohol. Chronic alcohol consumption results in Alcoholic Liver Diseases (ALD) like Cirrhosis, Alcoholic Hepatitis and Steatosis, and other serious health problems such as Alzheimer's disease, Hematological complications, Pancreatic problems, Sexual dysfunction and Infertility etc. Alcohol thus, has a very serious effect on the overall health of the addicted person.

The treatment of alcoholism involves different therapies besides medicines for comprehensive and smooth recovery of the person. The body psychotherapies deal with mind and body coordinated therapy covering different de-addiction techniques/processes available to combat the habit of alcoholism. Since this therapy involves combining of body and mind aspects in the healing process, the body-psychotherapies like Bio-energetic Analysis, Mindfulness, Hakomi and Rebirthing are explored and evaluated as possible alternatives in treating addiction. However, certain issues like expertise in such techniques, ethical issues, and adequate information about the addicted person should be kept in mind while using body-psychotherapies.

Prolonged use of alcohol increases the risks of Chronic Liver Disease, Fatty liver disease, Fibrosis, Cirrhosis, Alcoholic hepatitis etc. The liver aids in digestion of food, absorption of nutrients and detoxification, the probiotics meant for liver health might work as alternative therapy for alcoholism. Probiotics helps in intestinal immunity and also in epithelial viability. These are also beneficial in improving overall health and hence used as nutritional supplements. The damage to liver can be minimized with the use of probiotics.

The de-addiction therapies have different mode of operation. The chemical drugs might have side effect on patients, so the alternative medicines play a major role in de-addiction of an alcoholic without inducing side effects. The alternative medicines, mainly the herbs based Ayurvedic medicines, are highly useful in alcohol de-addiction therapies. Various herbs available in nature help in recovering the functioning of brain, nervous system, liver, digestive system and overall body health. Combination and controlled application of selected herbs help in complete recovery of the alcoholic patient. The different herbal drugs, formulations and combinations have varied impact on the body, so alternative therapy (Ayurveda and Herbal) should be followed in guidance of experts in field.

Psychopharmacotherapy is meant to develop strong psychological confidence along with treatment with drugs and when adopted it reflects positive results in psychosocial behaviour along with anticraving relapse maintenance. The Pharmacotherapy could be more effective in multimodal approach including psychological and social support. The section on Psychopharmacotherapy is a narration about many brain neurotransmitter systems (CNS) activities with various phases of addiction currently being used for pharmacotherapies and psychopharmacotherapies along with co-morbid disorders for treatment of alcoholism.

The management of alcohol and drug abuse go hand in hand with pharmacological and psychosocial approaches of the treatment. In the treatment of alcoholic person, the pharmacological (drug supplements) and psychosocial support (self-determination and family support) remain complementary to each other, and the best results have generally been obtained by a combined approach involving both approaches.

In overall, the culture, social norms and portrayal of norms impact the prevalence or cessation of alcoholism in particular place, state, nation. Heavy drinking impacts the vital organs of body particularly the liver. The therapies for alcoholism are wide, and comprehensive results are obtained with combined use of selected therapies. Alternative therapies might prove beneficial in complete recovering of addicted person.

Editors

Epilogue

To be or not to be an alcoholic?

Alcohol. There cannot be a better anachronism to describe the vagaries of nature of mankind as well as the laws of Nature!

Taboo. So say the Puritanists of society. Their viewpoint is justified forever because intake of alcohol is universally acknowledged as being the prime causative factor for all acts of crime. All criminal jurisprudence supports this truism of life.

Right. A right to liberate oneself with an innocuous exercise of intake of alcohol. So say the ones that enjoy this elixir of life. Undoubtedly so. A harmless time pass. As long as one consumes in one's own hearth or homestead. In moderate quantities a tonic to relax the nerves - as we all want to believe!

Break of harmony - at home and the entire neighbourhood. Here commences the concern of all right-thinking leaders of the World. Be they physicians, social activists, law-makers, makers and marketers of alcoholic beverages of all types, forms, brands...

Policy of any modern government to prohibit the sale of liquor in public places has been found to be ridden with holes, a dime a dozen.

To begin with, a certain State in the south of India has a tradition of offering freebies to poor electorate come election season. It was estimated to cost the exchequer a whopping twenty eight thousand crores of rupees! But, the clever ruler sourced this huge sum from an earning of thirty thousand crores of rupees through sale of alcohol by the State run outlets (including licensing system)! So, at the end of it all, there was still a savings of two thousand crores of rupees in the State kitty!!

Social studies reveal that it is the poor people who resort to alcohol and cheap liquor as a means of battling life's many challenges. The rich in any case enjoy their wine, liqueurs and consumption of any substance by them does not matter to pundits of economics, sociology or politics.

Having said this, it is pertinent to note that decadence of an individual starts when he turns an addict of alcohol. What was once a means to relaxation or 'social' habit soon gives way to the monsters inhabiting the being of the regular consumer. Thoughts gallop as race horses in the course but, all benumbed, bodily form turns as good as a corpse. Nervous wrecks emerge out of a lively being. Sensory organs go for a walk & no command of the brain is translated by an inebriated person! In short, a walking dead emerges from the one enslaved to the habit!

So arises the question: can society or a government, police the habitual drunkards?

Yes. Should- to check rise of crime rate. No. It is more of civic sense for both individuals of the community as well as the society as a whole which ought to self-regulate this strange addiction which only terminates real life activity. However, a comprehensive look must be had at the whole gamut of the alcoholism, alcohol-abuse, alcohol-driven lifestyle of modern day world around us.

Not fully in jest is it often said that an alcoholic is one who drinks more than his doctor!

Or, that fractures used to heal, even when there were no orthopaedic surgeons!

But, hindsight is a perfect science, so to speak. Hence, let us analyse the need to banish alcoholism from the lives of youngsters and future generations. For the good of society and for good of each and every human being.

Utopian ?

Yes. But, very essential.

It is not just societal problems that emanate from alcoholism but physical impairment of the consumer is bound to occur.

What is the use of existence? - ask the depressed people. They use this as a slogan to indulge in uninhibited, unrestricted, uncontrollable consumption of alcohol and indeed, they turn deadwood or live corpses, and life becomes wasted. A vegetative existence is the beginning of fall of all mankind. Unless there is growth, activity, development of the personality and society cumulatively, an insect's life appears to have greater purpose, meaning and interest for the Universe!

So, an ecosystem or the lifestyle adopted by each of us in the society of beasts, humans and trees determines the intolerance, acceptance or addiction to alcohol as a style statement of one's mental, economic & social quotient! .

The vulnerable, jobless and curious youngsters become victims of marketing wizards' bombardment of the fashionable page-3 cocktail circuit which is dubiously dubbed and propagated as ' up & flying' indication of success.

The horrendous tales of destruction and degenerated mindsets haunt families, generations and communities - worldwide!

Recovering from downslide is next to impossible. So, beware!

Even those who are addicted and enslaved to alcohol abuse often are heard to dissuade others in the society from falling prey to the 'bug of peg'!

A singular measure which can be taken by all of the society and the whole of the world is to ban prominent adverts with promiscuous looking images goading upon all to squander their wealth and often hard earned money on alcoholic beverages. After all, no one can stop you from taking the plunge into an evening or day of drinking splurge if you choose to, not to forget making a special mention of the drunken brawls that are often end-result of such uninhibited sessions. Daily bouts are but bound to result in criminal behaviour or premature death due to liver Cirrhosis and similar terminal conditions of health...

Such a regulation must be prescribed by every local government and one cannot await nor expect a 'western' World Health Organisation to dictate the good advice to the comity of nations across the globe.

Even more importantly, the State must impose heavy taxation on all activities related to alcohol, not just consumption.

This will act as a double-edged weapon: on one hand, it will fetch greater revenue for public welfare activities and on the other hand, this will help reduce the number of wanton consumers off this tantalising substance.

Reams and reams of paper have been utilised to drive better sense among populations of the country and in other parts of the world - both about the perils of drinking alcohol as a habit and multiple jeopardy which every consumer is facing. Many others have cried hoarse about spurious liquor and adulteration becoming an industry whenever prohibition policy takes shape.

There are little vociferous brigades who cite mythological names as Bacchus, Shiva & the wine dispensed as 'prasadam' in Catholic Churches after mass prayers!

Little do the dangers evaporate with such arguments of support to one's habits.

Hard core alcoholics soon convert into dipsomaniacs. Their existence revolves around the bottle, literally speaking. Medicinal effects vanish. Side effects adversely affect the bodily form. Firmness of grip and solidity of thought process gets diminished and the person soon turns into a puppet of the drops!

Violence soon forms a part of the psyche - both to the one deprived of alcohol and the ones who drown & drench themselves into alcohol in their waking hours. This permeates even in drawing rooms, bedrooms, not to speak of streets and only bedlam results. All is hell. Life becomes hell. Not just for the victim of this habit but to all those near & dear ones- be it parents, spouse, children, relatives, neighbouring people and total strangers!

Banal. Cannot ban it. Abandon it.

A perennial solution can only come from one's strength of character. This often is molded by one's religion, faith and upbringing.

Prescription and restrictions imposed by religious orders are seldom followed religiously even by the self-professed devout. So, is it destiny, karmic causes or is it absolutely a matter of one's decision to keep the tryst with destiny?

This is the signature tune of this universal document. Must one fall prey to an age-old habit? Or, should one stand strong, be confident and turn a Nelson's eye to this endangering if enticingly 'cool' habit?

The choice and answer determines your autobiography...

There are cultures where best of business moguls and preachers enjoy their drinks upon sunset but are up and fresh by sunrise to address a new fresh day's tasks in full senses. These are few & far – the people who enforce discipline even in such a cultivated or inherited habit.

And, then there are many more sane ones who indulge in buttermilk, curds and fresh fruit juices or simply water to thank the night for relieving them of a day's burden. They are otherwise as free thinking in mind and agile in bodily actions, day in & day out.

Sad is the case of those who fall prey and seek to indoctrinate rest of world into their Dracula like mission. They fall soon as dried leaves do, off a treetop !

It would not be out of place to present the fragile argument of those new breed of young Turks in business & profession who wail that unless social drinking is indulged in, they would lose out. To these folks, I say,' No, not at all. For, I have worked long hours and won largest of cases even of royal dynasties that forsake their cup of joy whenever an appointment with this lawyer was in place. You set the style of your work space. Do not succumb!'.

The long and short of it all, dear readers, is that alcoholism is a key determinant of your life: would you like to help it cut short your productive life or counter the itch & bug to clink glasses, for a happy, peaceful, long lifespan ?

To not fall prey, would enhance both the quality and term of one's lifetime...

– Pamarty Venkataramana
An Eminent Jurist & Poet from New Delhi, India

1

Is it the Personality or the Alcohol that Makes one an Addict?

Karishma*, Nisha Phakey* and Krishan Kumar*

Abstract

Alcohol is the most commonly abused substance creating serious medical, social & psychological problems. It exerts a toll on world health on a par with unsafe sex, measles and malaria and greater than tobaccos a total of more than three of quarters of a millions of deaths in 1990 was related to alcohol and 80% of it occurred in developing countries. It has been reported that alcohol was responsible for 6,34,800 deaths, 14.6 million years of life lost and 32.3 million disability adjusted years of life lost in 1998. The latter measure includes estimates of the impact of non-fatal alcohol caused injury and illness on general quality of life. Prevalence of alcohol problem varies across different cultural and social settings. Macro cultural influences values, beliefs and social role functions, local economy, customs and dietary habits, rapid social change and cultural stress do shape and dictate the way alcohol is used in human societies. There is strong evidence of several sorts for genetic predisposition, personality factors and learning to alcoholism. Here, in this chapter we are trying

* Institute of Mental Health, Pt. BD Sharma University of Health Sciences, Rohtak 124001. India.

to conceptualize all these issue for better understanding of this menace.

Keywords: Alcohol addiction, Personality, Big five personality traits, Type I Type II

INTRODUCTION

Addictive Behaviour

Addictions have plagued society throughout history, as is evident from the Greco-Roman philosopher's condemnation of excesses to our preoccupation with alcohol and drugs. The Oxford English Dictionary traces the term addiction to Roman law, under which addiction was a "formal giving over by sentence of court; hence a dedication of a person to a master." This notion of relinquishment of control by the addicted person is the central feature of many lay and professional definitions of the term. Traditionally, the term addiction has been used to identify self-destructive behaviours that include a pharmacological component. The most stringent application would limit the term addiction and the companion label of an addict to individuals with a physiological dependence on one or more illegal drugs. This definition usually includes a strong physiological craving, withdrawal symptom, and the need for more of the drug to get the same effect. (American Psychiatric Association, 1980)[1,2]

Types of Addictive Behavior

Drug Addiction: Addictive behavior, involving the pathological need for a substance. The most commonly used problem substances are the psychoactive drugs, those drugs that affect mental functioning: alcohol, barbiturates, minor tranquilizers, amphetamines, heroin and marijuana.

Other Addictive Behaviors: Many other behaviors are being increasingly recognized as being similar to the addictive behavior with regard to psychoactive substances.

Pathological Gambling: Pathological gambling is known as a disorder of impulse control (DSM-VI) but it can also be viewed as an addictive disorder. The compulsive gambler looses control over the behavior, denies that he has a problem, is easily depressed, and has a low self-image.

Computer/Internet Addiction: Over the past few years, with the increase in home computers and computer games, computer addicts or "hackers"

have begun to emerge. Compulsive computer interactors have been known to spend hours at the console without eating, bathing, or sleeping. When deprived of the computer, they go through withdrawal symptoms of irritability and anxiety. Much attention has been paid to the phenomenon of Internet Addiction, conceived of as a compulsive behavior, or craving for connectedness, or perhaps even a manifestation of transference or a reflection of object relations, or need-fulfillment.

Sexual Addiction: The concept of compulsive sexual behavior, or sex addiction, developed over the past two decades to describe persons who compulsively seek out sexual experiences and whose behavior becomes impaired if they cannot gratify their sexual impulses. Here the person's entire life revolves around sex-seeking behavior and activities, who spends an excessive amount of time in such behavior, and who often tries to stop such behavior but cannot do so.

Alcohol Addiction

The attraction of man to alcohol has existed throughout history. Countless fruits have produced, by countless techniques, many forms of alcoholic beverages. Always, too much of this good thing led to excess and inebriety, and the struggle within society for and against the use of alcohol was waged.[3] But what is that has drawn mankind to alcoholism, many factors affect the decision to drink, the development of temporary alcohol-related difficulties, and the development of alcohol dependence.[4] The initiation of alcohol intake and maintenance depends on many factors including heredity, environment and social (such as adverse experiences during childhood, mental illness, discord, violence, stressful family life, peer pressure and psychological complications), pharmacology of the drug and the personality of the individual.[5,6]

The ICD-10 Classification of Mental and Behavioural Disorders Criteria for alcohol dependance:-

A definite diagnosis of dependence should usually be made only if three or more of the following have been present together at some time during the previous year:

(*a*) a strong desire or sense of compulsion to take the substance;

(*b*) difficulties in controlling substance-taking behaviour in terms of its onset, termination, or levels of use;

(*c*) a (physiological withdrawal state) when substance use has ceased or been reduced, as evidenced by: the characteristic withdrawal syndrome for the substance; or use of the same (or a closely related) substance with the intention of relieving or avoiding withdrawal symptoms;

(*d*) evidence of tolerance, such that increased doses of the psychoactive substance are required in order to achieve effects originally produced by lower doses (clear examples of this are found in alcohol- and opiate-dependent individuals who may take daily doses sufficient to incapacitate or kill non tolerant users);

(*e*) progressive neglect of alternative pleasures or interests because of psychoactive substance use, increased amount of time necessary to obtain or take the substance or to recover from its effects;

(*f*) persisting with substance use despite clear evidence of overtly harmful consequences, such as harm to the liver through excessive drinking, depressive mood states consequent to periods of heavy substance use, or drug-related impairment of cognitive functioning; efforts should be made to determine that the user was actually, or could be expected to be, aware of the nature and extent of the harm.[7]

ETIOLOGY

Genetics

There is strong evidence of several sorts for genetic predisposition to alcoholism. Family attitudes toward drinking, modeling, maladaptive efforts to cope with the pain and trauma of growing up in an alcoholic family, identification with the aggressor, and social learning have all been implicated. All of these factors play a role, but current thinking leans toward genetic transmission of vulnerability as a primary causal element running the in families.[5] Approximately 60 percent of the people who are at risk for alcohol use disorders are influenced by specific genes which affects the vulnerability toward alcoholism. Although, as is true of most genetically influenced traits, multiple genes contribute to each of these characteristics.[4]

Learning Theories

The behavioral models of substance use disorder postulate that substance use behavior is a result of learning and maintained through as follows:

(*i*) **Classical conditioning:** Through this learning process the individual is thought to facilitate development of a drinking or drug problems through pairing of conditioned stimuli (CS) such as particular sites of use or people and the un-conditioning stimuli (UCS: Alcohol or Drugs), the result being a conditioned response (CR), or conditioned craving.[8]

(*ii*) **Operant conditioning:** This principle suggests that the positive reinforcing effect of alcohol and drugs as social reinforcers, and to the avoidance or cessation of withdrawal symptoms.

(*iii*) **Social learning theory:** Drinking behavior is governed by principle of learning, cognition and reinforcement (Bandura,1969). The social learning theory suggests that drinking as a social behavior is acquired and maintained by modeling, social reinforcement, and the anticipated effects of alcohol and physical dependence.[9]

(*iv*) **Expectancy theory:** The importance of cognitive factors in the initiation and maintenance of drinking behavior is central to expectancy model (Blane and Leonard, 1987). Individual's drinking is determined by his alcohol expectancies rather than by its mere pharmacological effects.[10]

(*v*) **Tension reduction hypothesis:** This hypothesis suggests alcohol is consumed to achieve tension reduction.[11]

Personality

As heredity and learning models failed to establish any concrete link causing alcohol addiction, the question arised if there is an 'alcoholic personality'. A myriad number of researchers have tried to establish the link between personality and alcohol addiction.

Personality is the dynamic organization within the individual of those psychophysical systems that determines his characteristic behavior and thought.[12]

Psychodynamic Theories

By the twentieth century, explanations for alcoholism and addiction were regularly put forward by psychiatry and psychoanalysis. The very first psychoanalytic formulations received their impetus from Freud. He believed that alcoholism was the result of strong oral influences in childhood. Alcohol provides a mood alteration and consequent redirection of thought processes, providing the impetus for regressive levels of thinking and for achieving gratification from thinking unrelated to logic. Alcohol provides an escape from reality.

Mellinger advanced a self destructive drive as the prime component of alcoholism. Addiction was considered the means used by those persons who unconsciously have a powerful urge to destroy themselves, an urge derived from guilt associated with the child's anger toward his parents, whose behavior during childhood frustrated his need for oral gratification. He contended that the conflict involves the child's intense rage, in which he wishes to destroy his parents yet fears loosing them. Later in life, alcohol becomes the means to achieve gratification and revenge: hostility experienced through antisocial behavior while under the influence of alcohol and resultant punishment when sober to alleviate guilt. Therefore, he sees alcoholism as a form of chronic suicide.

Adler attributed the cause of addiction to powerful feelings of inferiority related to a perpetual state of insecurity and a desire to escape responsibility. An alcoholic addiction may be predicted by many traits for example: by marked shyness, a preference for isolation, impatience, irritability, anxiety, depression, hypersensitivity and sexual inadequacy. He incriminated over indulgence leading to an inability to face the frustration of adulthood, and the subsequent use of alcohol as a method of countering the demands of society.[3]

David McClelland worked on the relationship of the need for power and alcoholism.[13] Frustrated ambitions may play a role in the development of an alcoholic problem. He suggests that alcoholic may have an enhanced need for power but is inadequate to achieve his goals. He uses alcohol because it gives him a sense of release and of power and feelings of achievement.[3]

Till the decades of 1930s and 1940s, abundant research was pursued in looking for an 'alcoholic personality' but by the 1950s critical reviews of the literature on alcoholism reported that there was no consistent evidence for a distinct alcoholic personality. The Alcoholics Subcommittee of the World Health Organization (WHO) discouraged the search for an alcoholic personality. This decline in the view of personality predicting alcohol abuse was short lived and within a couple of year's research in this context started resurfacing.[14]

E.M. Jellinek's Classification

Though it was short lived, in 1960s E.M. Jellinek attempted to devise a new classification of alcoholic persons in terms of "Alpha, Beta, Gamma,

Delta and Epsilon alcoholism". Alpha alcoholism was described as a purely psychological continual reliance on the effect of alcohol to relieve bodily or emotional pain. Although society may view the drinking as beyond the norm because the time, place, amount and effect are beyond the implied conventions, drinking in this group does not lead to uncontrolled drinking or an inability to abstain. Most consequences of the drinking pattern involve the family, financial or work crisis, lower productivity and perhaps nutritional deficiencies.

Alpha alcoholism is viewed not as disease entity per se but as a medicinal use of alcohol, taken to deal symptomatically with underlying pathological discomfort. He admitted that often there is progression to more serious drinking patterns and he further complicated his definition by noting that alpha alcoholism can often be referred to as "problem drinking" or as impliening a physical dependence on alcohol.

"Beta alcoholism" represents as the form of alcoholism where in physical complications often occur, but there is no physical or psychological dependence on alcohol.

"Gamma alcoholism" represents the most serious form of alcoholism. Here is seen increased tissue tolerance to alcohol, withdrawal symptoms and loss of control. It also indicates definite progression from psychological to physical dependence associated with marked behavioural alterations.

"Delta alcoholism" is like gamma alcoholism, except that the delta alcoholic person can't refrain from partaking of alcohol even for a day or two.

However, this classification system failed to make its mark and is not widely used.[3]

With the rise of poly drug dependence in the 7th decade, researchers observed that alcoholics who also abused other drugs had different personality characteristics from those who did not and these characteristics had implications for treatment. Such individuals were noted to be younger, more impulsive, disinhibited and extroverted, and seemed to do poorly in treatment programs designed to help more pure alcoholics. By the 1980's new models were put forward to measure personality in alcoholics, which can be roughly divided into two models. The first model focuses on personality psychopathology conceptualized as personality disorders. The majority of studies on alcoholism centre on antisocial personality disorder and its predecessor, conduct disorder. The second focuses on normally distributed personality measures. Several dimensional models have been promoted as comprehensive accounts of the major dimensions underlying adult personality.[14]

Antisocial Personality Disorder

Antisocial personality disorder is based on evidence of multiple severe antisocial behaviors beginning before the age of 15 as conduct disorder and continuing into adulthood. People with antisocial personality disorder are likely to be impulsive, violent, risk takers who do not easily learn or benefit from punishment. Probably as a reflection of these characteristics, 80 percent or more of people with antisocial personality disorder develop severe alcohol problems and are more likely than the average alcohol-dependent person to have a coexisting drug diagnosis, to be violent, to discontinue treatment prematurely, and to have a relatively poor prognosis. Other than antisocial personality disorder, high rates of comobridity of alcoholism has also been found with borderline personality disorder.[4,14,15,16]

Dimensional Models

In the field of alcoholism the most studied dimensional models so far have been Eysenck's big three model, Costa and McCrae Big Five Model and Cloninger's Type I and Type II alcoholism.[14,17]

Hans Eysenck's Big Three Model

The big three traits of Hans Eysenck's Big Three model are extraversion (*e.g.*, sensation seeking, assertiveness, sociability, dominance, venturesomeness), neuroticism (*e.g.*, anxiousness, depressiveness, guilt, low self-esteem), and psychoticism (*e.g.*, aggressiveness, impulsivity, tough-mindedness, creativity, antisociality). Although extraversion, neuroticism, and psychoticism may represent independent risk factors for alcohol abuse or dependence, they may co-occur and increase the risk for the development of alcohol-related problems.[18]

The Big Five Personality Traits

These are the best accepted and most commonly used model of personality. The five factors are as follows:

Extroversion: This dimension contrasts such traits as sociable, outgoing, talkative, assertive, persuasive, decisive, and active with more introverted traits such as withdrawn, quiet, passive, retiring and reserved.

Neuroticism: People high on neuroticism are prone to emotional instability. They tend to experience negative emotions and to be moody, irritable, nervous, and inclined to worry. This dimension differentiates people who are anxious, excitable, and easily distressed from those who are emotionally stable and thus calm, even-tempered, easygoing, and relaxed.

Conscientiousness: This dimension differentiates the individuals who are dependable, organized, reliable, responsible, thorough, hard-working, and persevering from those who are undependable, unorganized, impulsive, reliable, irresponsible, careless, negligent, and laze.

Agreeableness: This dimension is composed of a collection of traits that range from compassion to antagonism toward others. A person high on Agreeableness would be a pleasant person, who is good-natured, warm, sympathetic, and cooperative, one low on Agreeableness would tend to be unfriendly, unpleasant, aggressive, argumentative, cold, even hostile and vindictive.

Openness to Experience: This dimension contrasts individuals who seek out varied experiences and who are imaginative, intellectually curious, and broad-minded with those who are concrete-minded & practical and whose interests are narrow. Researchers have found that being high on Openness to Experience is a requirement for creative accomplishment.

NEO-PIR or NEO FFI are among the most frequently used measures to assess the big five traits.[12]

In the recent past many research studies with the aim of finding relations between the Big-Five personality domains and motivations for drinking alcohol were carried out. Research findings are suggestive that persons having been addicted to alcohol (present or past) have a high level of "Neuroticism", a low "Agreeableness" and a low level of "Conscientiousness", contrary to those who have never been addicted to alcohol. Among the patients with a past or present diagnosis of alcohol abuse, researchers found a low score on facets "trust", "achievement striving", "self-discipline" and "dutifulness" and a high score on "impulsiveness", "vulnerability", and "excitement-seeking".[19,20,21,22,23]

Type I and Type II Alcoholism

Cloninger's typology resulted from a study of alcoholism and other relevant characteristics in a large number of Swedish adoptees and their biological and adoptive parents. This typology distinguishes alcoholics according to the inheritance patterns of their alcoholism (i.e., whether the involved genes are passed on primarily from father to son or from both parents to both sons and daughters) and the relative contributions of genetic and environmental factors to the individual's susceptibility for developing the disease. The two subtypes identified are called type I (milieu-limited) and type called type II (male-limited). Type I alcoholism affects both men and women, requires the presence of a genetic as well as an environmental predisposition, commences later in life after years of heavy drinking, and can take on either a mild or severe form. Type II alcoholism, in contrast, affects mainly sons of male alcoholics, is influenced only weakly by environmental factors, often begins during adolescence or early adulthood, is characterized by moderate severity, and usually is associated with criminal behavior. Gradually, researchers investigated whether reproducible differences in personality traits existed between type I and type II alcoholics. These analyses identified three heritable personality traits that could describe the prototypical characteristics of both alcoholism subtypes: harm avoidance, novelty seeking, and reward dependence. The term "harm avoidance" describes whether a person is cautious, apprehensive, pessimistic, and inhibited (i.e., high harm avoidance) or confident, relaxed, optimistic, and uninhibited (i.e., low harm avoidance). People with high novelty seeking traits are impulsive, exploratory, and distractible, whereas people with low novelty seeking traits are rigid, reflective, and attentive to detail. Finally, a high reward dependence describes subjects who are eager to help others, emotionally dependent, sentimental, and sensitive to social cues, whereas subjects with low reward dependence are socially detached, emotionally cool, practical, and tough minded. A myriad number of studies have demonstrated that type I alcoholics frequently exhibited high harm avoidance, low novelty seeking, and high reward dependence personality characteristics indicating high levels of anxiety. Type II alcoholics often exhibited a reverse personality profile, with low harm avoidance, high novelty seeking, and low reward dependence. This combination of traits also describes people with antisocial personality disorder (ASPD) and is consistent with findings that type II alcoholics frequently suffer from ASPD.[24]

A very similar typology was given by T. F Babor. His type A alcohol dependence is characterized by late onset, few childhood risk factors, relatively mild dependence, few alcohol related problems, and little psychopathology. Type B on the other hand is characterized by many childhood risk factors, severe dependance, and much psychopathology, a strong family history of alcohol abuse, an early onset of alcohol related problems, frequent polysubstance abuse, along history of alcohol treatment and a lot of severe life stresses.[25]

CONCLUSION

Historians have proved that intentionally fermented beverages have existed since centuries, and psychologists have tried to understand the causality of mankind's bend towards alcoholism since almost a century. Various etiological factors contribute to it including psychological, genetic, learning and personality of the individual. A myriad number of personality theories and typologies have been formulated to establish if it's the personality that determines the nature of alcohol use in the individual. The substantial part of the innumerable studies have correlated the high level of neuroticism, a low level of conscientiousness, impulsiveness, high level of novelty-seeking and antisocial traits with alcohol addiction.

REFERENCES

1. Kranzler, R.H. Li, T. Kai. What is addiction. *Alcohol Res Health*. **2008**, 31(2), 93-95.
2. C.C. Diclemente . Addiction and Change: How Addictions Develop and Addicted People Recover, Guilford Press: New York, **2003**.
3. M.A. Freedman, I.H. Kaplan . Comprehensive Textbook of Psychiatry. Indian Edition. Williams &Wilkins: Calcutta, **1967**.
4. B.J. Sadock, V.A. Sadock, P. Ruiz. Kaplan & Sadock's Comprehensive Textbook of Psychiatry.9thed.Lippincott Williams & Wilkins: Philadelphia, **2009**.
5. D. Brizer, R. Castaneda. Clinical addiction psychiatry. Cambridge University Press: New York, **2010**.
6. C. Dubey, M. Arora, S. Gupta, B. Kumar. Five factor correlates: a comparison of substance abusers and non-substance abusers. *J. Ind. Acad. Appl. Psychol.*, **2010**, 36, 107-114.
7. World Health Organisation ICD-10, International Statistical Classification of Diseases and Related Health Problems, 10th Revision: Geneva, **1992**, 75-76.

8. A. Wikler. Dynamics of drug dependence: Implications of a conditioning theory or research and treatment. *Arch Gen Psychiatry*. **1973**, 28(5), 611-66.
9. A. Bandura. Principles of Behavior Modification. Holt: Rinehart& Winston: New York, 1969.
10. H.T. Blane, K.E. Leonard. Introduction. In: Psychological Theories of Drinking and Alcoholism. The Guilford Press: New York, 1987.
11. J.J. Conger. Alcoholism: Theory, problem and challenge. II. Reinforcement theory and the dynamics of alcoholism. Q.J. Stud. Alcohol. 1956, 17, 296-305.
12. S.E. Wood, E.G. Wood, D. Boyd. The World of Psychology. Pearson: New York, 2013.
13. D.C. McClelland, W.N. Davis, Kalin, E.Wanner. The drinking man.Free Press: New York, 1972.
14. T.R. Mulder Alcoholism and personality. *AustN Z J Psychiatry*. **2002**, 36(1), 44–52.
15. K.J. Sher, T.J. Trull. Personality and disinhibitory psychopathology: alcoholism and antisocial personality disorder. *J Abnorm Psychol*. **1994**, 103, 92–102.
16. R. Verheul. Co-morbidity of personality disorders in individuals with substance use disorders. *Eur Psychiatry*. **2001**, 16(5), 274–282.
17. J.M. Malouff, B.E. Thorsteinsson, E.S. Rooke, S.N. Schutte. Alcohol involvement and the five-factor model of personality: a meta-analysis. *J drug educ*. **2007**, 37(3), 277-294.
18. K.R. Brooner, D. Templer, S.D. Svikis, C. Schmidt, Monopolis. Dimensions of alcoholism: a multivariate analysis. *Journal of studies on alcohol*. **1990**, 51, 77-81.
19. N. Lackner, H.M. Unterrainer, A.C. Neubauer. Differences in Big Five Personality Traits Between Alcohol and Polydrug Abusers: Implications for Treatment in the Therapeutic Community. *Int. J. Mental Health and Addiction*. **2013**, 11, 682-692.
20. E.D. Martin, K.J. Sher. Family History of Alcoholism, Alcohol Use Disorders and the Five-Factor Model of Personality. *J Stud Alcohol*. **1994**, 55, 81-90.
21. S. Chaudhary, S.K. Das, B. Ukil. Psychological assessment of alcoholism in males. *Ind. J. Psychiatry*. **2006**, 48, 114–117.
22. K. Flory, D. Lyman, R. Milich, C. Leukefeld, R. Clayton. The relations among personality, symptoms of alcohol and marijuana abuse, and symptoms of comorbid psychopathology: results from a community sample. *ExpClinPsychophamacol*. **2002**, 10, 425-34.

23. M.A. Ruiz, A.L. Pincus, K.A. Dickinson. NEO PI-R predictors of alcohol use and alcohol-related problems. *J Pers Assess.* **2003**, 81, 226-36.

24. C.R. Cloninger, S. Sören, B. Michael. Type-I and Type-II Alcoholism: An Update. *Alcohol Health and Research.* **1996**, 20, 18-23.

25. T.F. Babor, M. Hofmann, F.K. Delboca, V. Hesselbrock, R.E. Meyer, Z.S. Dolinsky, B.Rounsaville. Types of alcoholics: I. Evidence for an empirically derived typology based on indicators of vulnerability and severity. *Archives of General Psychiatry*. **1992**, 49, 599–608.

Editors' Note

Alcoholism may have many causes and people with certain personality are more prone to it. Factors such as genetics, childhood influences, antisocial behavior, and personality traits also contribute towards menance of alcoholism in individuals. Personality traits like extroversion, neuroticism, conscientiousness, agreeableness and openness to experience influence the addiction in individuals. Cultural values, beliefs and childhood experiences govern thought process which is indirectly related to earlier stages of alcohol addiction. Family history and life stress have implications on individual/s susceptibility to alcohol addiction.

❑❑❑

2

Impact of Alcohol on Family Functioning

Narendra Kumar Singh* and Dipanjan Bhattacharjee*

Abstract

Alcoholism has now been conceptualized as a chronic, progressive, and often fatal disease. Previously alcoholism was understood as a form of 'social deviation'. It is a primary disorder and not a symptom of other diseases or emotional problems. The formal term of consumable alcohol is 'ethanol' or 'ethyl alcohol'. Ethanol or ethyl alcohol is the predominant alcohol in alcoholic beverages. Alcohol causes very significant impact of almost all types of cells and tissues in human body, including those in the central nervous system. Prolonged alcohol consumption causes plethora of changes in the nervous system of the consuming individuals. Dependence to alcoholic beverages leads to significant damages to the both Central and Peripheral Nervous Systems and very often those damages could pose to be irreversible in nature. Alcohol consumption can have negative impacts in all domains of a person's life that is physical, social, financial and familial. The impact of alcohol on familial aspects has been widely evaluated by many researchers in the past. In this chapter, consequences of chronic alcoholism on the structure and function of families have been discussed.

Keywords: Alcoholism, Family, Impact Analysis, Intervention.

* Department of Psychiatric Social Work, Central Institute of Psychiatry, Kanke, Ranchi, Jharkhand, India.

INTRODUCTION

Alcoholism is a chronic, progressive, and often fatal disease. It is a primary disorder and not a symptom of other diseases or emotional problems. The chemistry of alcohol allows it to affect nearly every type of cell in the body, including those in the central nervous system. After prolonged exposure to alcohol, the brain adapts to the changes alcohol makes and becomes dependent on it.

Prolong alcohol consumption causes negative impacts on almost every possible sphere of one's life, *e.g.* physical, psychological, social, financial and family. The impact of alcohol on family has been widely studied. Alcohol dependence causes wide-scale damage to every areas and faculties of family system. Alcoholism has the enduring negative impacts on family's both structure and function. Areas like marital or spousal relationship, intra-family interpersonal relationship, and family's role performance both at individual and general levels, family's economic affairs, child raising and parenting functions, interactions with neighbourhood, community and larger social agencies and institutions are greatly affected by alcoholism. Alcoholism is associated with the development of coercive relationship between the partners which often tends to end up in termination of marriage in most undesirable manner.[1] In United States, alcohol addiction has been found to be the chief causal factor in nearly 80% of violent family incidents and in Britain the figure is approximately 75%.[1] Undesirable incidents like child abuse and neglect are quite common in families with habitual alcohol users.[1,2] The relationship between the family and alcoholism can be explained by two mutually divergent rationales, *e.g. firstly,* 'alcoholism has very strong genetic or familial components, since very often alcohol addiction runs through multiple generations of the family system' and *secondly,* 'alcoholism severely impairs family functions and relationship trajectories'. It is a known fact that alcoholism increases the risk of undesirable consequences like 'domestic violence', 'marital disharmony', 'sexual and physical abuse', 'violence on spouse/partner', 'child abuse and neglect', 'financial hardships', 'undercare of family members or inadequate fulfilment of their needs', 'occupational problems', 'homelessness' and 'involvement in criminal and antisocial activities' and all those issues have direct implications on families.[3-5]

Empirical observations suggested that in affected families alcohol become prime center around which all family interaction and dynamics revolve.

This kind of family only seeks temporary stability by grossly affecting permanent stability.[6] Thus the development and organization of family gets impaired as consequence of alcoholism.[7] The economic, psychological, emotional, and physical consequences of alcoholism intensify further conflict and problems where family members become undicisive towards their capacity to choose appropriate coping strategy.[8] Such families usually form rigid external boundaries with diffused and enmeshed internal interpersonal boundaries[9]. If family organization and dynamics are settled well on alcoholism then there is danger of transmission of alcoholism to coming generation as family settlement to alcoholism become part of family tradition and family rituals.[10]

ALCOHOLISM AND FAMILY DYNAMICS

Drug addiction and alcoholism can be viewed as a symptom of a dysfunctional family system in which the addicted person emerges as the identified patient of the system. The addiction and associated behaviors evolve within the family and become an integral part of that system, helping to define roles, boundaries, and subsystem. The dynamic relationship between family and alcoholism can be holistically explained by applying the renowned *'Family Systems Model'*. The Family Systems Model suggests alcohol can operate as an important factor in maintaining the family homeostasis or equilibrium process. As per family systems theory, family functions as an organized system in encouraging, reinforcing, and finally sustaining the alcohol-seeking behaviour in addicted members.[11-14] Majority of the past studies on families of alcohol addicts suggested two mutually divergent observations regarding the relationship between parents and their addicted offspring, (a) one parent tends to become supportive to addictive behavior or intensely involves with the addicted person; (b) another parent adopts the punitive stance—here he or she tries to be critical to the addicted person or tries to distance him or herself from the addicted person. The common observation suggests that the over involved indulgent or overprotective parent happens to be the opposite sex from the abuser. This over involvement may even culminate to the most undesirable consequence like 'incest'. Development of incestuous relationship can occur if the addicted person is the female child. Very often, abusing offspring may even serve a function for the parents, either as a medium for their communication, or as a person who creates massive disruption in the communication process of the family. Furthermore, the abuser may adopt the *"sick-role"* status in the family with the aim to assume a childlike position and get the continuous attention from parents. In case of adolescent onset alcohol addiction, parents tend to develop a sense of fear and panic of losing their adolescent child to outsiders, since their addicted child tends to mix with his social network more where he gets addictive substances as well as the company of addicts. This way, the family sticks at this particular developmental stage and a chronic, repetitive process tends to set in which is characterized by the features like 'individuation', 'growing up', and 'separation of the addicted child from the family in undesirable manner'. Nearly four decades back, Stanton *et.al*[15] identified some distinctive features of the families with alcohol and other psychoactive substances addicts. Those were: (a) Higher chances of multigenerational chemical dependency—particularly alcohol among males—as well as other addiction-like behaviours like gambling and watching television. Those practices tend to diffuse in multiple generations of the family system because of modeling or imitating addictive behavior by children; children adopt those behaviours from their addicted elders and reckon those maladaptive behaviours as the 'traditions of the family'; (b) In those families more primitive and direct expression of conflict, with quite overt (versus covert) alliances could be seen. This particular phenomenon occurs between the addict and his/her overinvolved parent; (c) Addict parents' behaviour is very often expressed as *"conspicuously unschizophrenic"* in quality; (d) Addicted individuals develop an alcohol or drug-centric sub-culture which includes his/her peer groups or people with who they take addictive substances. In those sub-cultures they tend to dissociate themselves from family conflict—and seek the illusory independence or autonomy; (e) Mothers of those addicted individuals tend to develop a "symbiotic" child rearing practices further into the life of the child; (f) In those families preponderance of death themes characterized by premature, unexpected, or untimely deaths could be seen; (g) The symptom of addiction facilitates a form of "pseudo-individuation" at multiple levels, extending from the individual-pharmacological level to that of the drug subculture; (h) Families having the history of migration harbor higher risk of afflicting alcohol and other substance addiction owing to acculturation related stress and less acceptance in the host culture or getting hostile treatment in the host society.

Pattison & Kaufman[8] described three distinct family interaction patterns. The first is the *Functional Family System*; it is the kind of family where some members consume alcohol. These families usually adapted their family functions and are responsive to external change. A minimum of overt conflict exists and the focus of the family is likely on the alcoholic. Here alcoholism is way of coping with personal and social stress and most of time alcohol consumption is taken place away from home. This kind of families represents early phases of alcoholism but the deterioration comes with passing time.

The second family type is the *Neurotic Enmeshed Family System*, here the behaviour of entire family is focused on alcohol. In these families, practice of alcohol consumption dysregulate the normal family routine, here changes comes in role structuring, various sorts of interpersonal conflicts arises and crisis for adaptation emerges, in later stages interpersonal conflicts leads to further deterioration in the system.

A third pattern is the *Disintegrated Family System* or the separated family. Here progressive biopsychosocial deterioration and family instability leads to a diffuse the families boundaries and adversely fragmented the family system. Such kinds of families initially shows apparently better adjustment but in later stages family collapses.

Steinglass[7] added further explanation in the above-mentioned family phenomenon described by Pattison & Kaufman[8]. He applied the mechanism of *morphostatic force* (family homeostatic resistance to change and regulatory mechanisms that maintain stability) and a *morphogenic force* (family reorganization associated with growth, change, or development).

Thus, it is evident that alcoholism and family functioning have relationship of cause and effect. At one stage, family problems and conflict serve to evoke, support, and maintain drinking behaviour.[16] On the other hand alcoholism can be a coping mechanism for the alcoholic and the family to deal with dysfunctional patterns and relationships. And in this way be a symptom of pathological family styles, rules, and patterns of alcohol use.[10] Families' responses to alcoholism can roughly be divided into four phases. These are called reactive, active, alternative and family unity phases. These phases have distinctive features and characteristics. Nonetheless, these phases may not be expressed and evolved in all alcoholic families uniformly. Many families tend to remain in the first phase and never reach the fourth state of sobriety and family growth. The reactive phase is characterized by the behaviour of non-alcoholic family members reacting to the alcoholic's behavior. At this phase, most family members tend to be overly cautious in their behavioural expressions, because their primary target at this phase is to avoid further worsening of the existing problems of alcoholism. However, by being reactive, they keep on constantly adapting their behaviour for reconciling the unhealthy family situation. At this phase, three typical family characteristics can be observed, such as: family denial, coping strategies, and social disengagement. The next phase is *'Active Phase'*. At this phase family members start to show some potential actions. At this phase, rather than being passive to the effects on themselves from alcoholism, they begin to take an active interest in themselves. Family members no longer perceive themselves as totally under the alcoholic's control, and they attempt to gain some control over their own lives. The next phase is *'Alternative Phase'*. This phase sets in when all other options have failed to create any meaningful impact on the family situation or control the alcohol addiction. At this phase family members have to tackle the most painful situation, *i.e.* whether to stay with the addicted person or dissociate him from the other family members or let the addicted person know that unless he control himself he will not be supported or cared in the family and he should desert himself from others. Because other family members see this is only the viable alternative to survive alcoholism. It is not necessary that a family should undergo both of the previous phases. Some families will go directly from the reactive phase into the alternative phase, while some others will attempt the active phase before making the final decision to separate. This phase has some distinctive characteristics, *e.g.* polarization, separation, change, and family re-organization. The final phase is *'Family Unity Phase'*. However, not all families reach at this stage because of the continuation of alcoholism. There are no definitive progressive patterns that end up to the unity phase. Some families will proceed directly from phase one to phase four, others will go through the first two phases and then onto four, and still others may go through all the phases on their way to family unity. When they reach at this phase they may face three concerns which are characteristic of this phase: sobriety, the "dry drunk," and family growth.[17-20]

IMPACT OF CHRONIC ALCOHOLISM ON VARIOUS FACETS OF THE FAMILY

Dependence to alcohol and other forms of psychoactive substances has now been unanimously accepted as a form of disease which has myriad physiological, psychological, social and cultural antecedents. Alcoholism has also been regarded a problem with very high level of affinity to various societal and family/community centric components. Several empirical research studies have shown that alcoholism could cause enduring changes or alterations in numerous family related structures and functions. Very often those changes are found to be negatively operational in the larger family systems.

ALCOHOLISM AND EMOTIONAL CLIMATE IN THE FAMILY SYSTEM

Presence of optimal emotional climate is an important prerequisite of a normal family system. Family cohesion can be understood as the *"emotional bonding that family members have toward one another"*.[21] Family cohesion has also been understood as the support, affection, and sense of caring family members keep for one another.[22] The variable of family cohesion is deeply influenced by several factors like 'the quality of emotional bonding exiting among members', 'intra-family and inter-family boundaries', 'patterns of coalitions exiting in the family system', 'time, space, friends, decision-making, and interests and recreation accepted and adored in the family system', etc. To be called as optimal emotional climate, the family system should have optimal presence for all those factors. Research shows that, families with addiction problem usually experience family disruption,[23-24] family violence,[25-27] loss of employment and financial instability,[24, 28] marital breakdown,[29] and physical and psychological abuse.[25,27,30] Presence of those problems eventually wrecks the core of the family system and processes and leads to development of disharmonious relationship among members. As per Pattison and Kaufman[8] alcoholism in the long run not only creates massive disturbances in the family but also disable family members' ability to see and interpret the normal family functions and structure. Because of enduring alcoholism, family members wrongfully alter their behavioural actions and practices to get accustomed with the maladaptive practice of their addicted relative. Family members adopt the maladaptive behavioural pattern to evade instances like 'development of family turmoil or conflicts'. But they indirectly or even directly promote the dysfunctional behavioural pattern in the family and ultimately that dysfunctional family system promotes, and maintains the alcoholism. Few authors referred alcoholism as family illness, because alcoholism has high degree of familial influence or propensity to run across many generations.[31, 32] Family studies show that first-degree relatives of alcoholics have three to five times higher likelihood to become addicts than the general population.[32,33] According to Liepman *et al*[34] the family functioning in major areas of alcohol-involved couples tends to be biphasic in nature, since it oscillates between the drinking and abstinent periods. It suggests that whenever addicted members keep sobriety or abstinent then the quality of family functions tends to become normal and when the problem of addiction goes up, functions of the family tend to decline. Frankenstein *et al*[35] during the abstinence period the nonalcoholic spouse have the onus in the family interaction pattern as well as emotional climate of the family. The quality of interpersonal relationship as well as emotional transactions between the couples become more negative (*e.g.*, criticized, blamed) during the active drinking phase.[36-38] Presence of high family cohesion could operate as protecting factor to youths against substance addiction.[39] Balanced or normal family is understood as the facilitator optimal care and affection to their members and those families are also believed to be functioning more effectively while dealing with substance addiction or preventing the development of addiction problem within the family system. These families try to provide adequate space for each individual member which is coupled with relentless support and care for family members.[40] Cropping up of alcohol use has been found to be a usual phenomenon among families that are non-cohesive or overly-cohesive.[40]

ALCOHOLISM AND FAMILY'S COMMUNICATION PATTERN

Renowned Argentina born US Psychiatrist and Family Theorist Salvador Minuchin[41] once stated that communication strategies can become erroneous because of the presence of stereotyped patterns of interaction among members. Overly presence of this type of communication can reduce the degree of openness in a family system. This openness is a prerequisite thing for optimal development of a family system. As per Minuchin, those families could become closed systems in the long run and the members individually and family as a whole will not have the ability to produce and use coping mechanisms in normal fashion. Such kinds of families are usually affected by chronic problem like alcohol and substance addiction and/or psychiatric disorders.[41] Haverfield *et al*[42] found that communication pattern in families of alcohol addicted individuals is generally faulty and inadequate. In those families some prototype communicational patterns are seen, thus: (a) aggressive communication (*e.g.*, presence of increase conflict, tense communication, and secretive slandering among members);

(b) protective communication (*e.g.*, existence of superficiality, limited or indirect communication, and sober parent buffering in the family); (c) adaptive communication (*e.g.*, insistence to functional communication among members); and, (d) inconsistent communication (*e.g.*, family members involvement in struggles over power and control, frequent mood fluctuation while interactions). Presence of alcohol addiction in family's guiding force or leadership or decision making figures like parents (either one or both parents) could cause enormous impact on the communicational and interpersonal interaction patterns of the family. Parental alcoholism negatively affects several dimensions of family functioning which have very close link with communication system of the family (*i.e.*, frequent occurrences of conflict and problems in expressing the positive feelings, emotionality, affection and cohesion).[43,44] According to Black[45] in alcoholic families, children are given the understanding that they should not discuss anything wrong about their alcohol addicted parent's(s) behaviour and activity. Because, this may cause hamper in the family functions further. In those families very often children are punished if they do not communicate as per the directives of parents and parents use communication to control the behaviour of their children. Ritchie and Fitzpatrick[46] defined family communication as: *'The family communication environment is a set of norms governing the tradeoff between informational and relational objectives of communication'*. These authors also talked about two dimensions of family communication, such as 'conversation orientation' (from 'concept orientation') and to 'conformity orientation' (from 'socio-orientation'). In conversation-oriented families provide the necessary environment and space to their children for developing the ability to recognize, understand and manage their own and others' emotions. Oppositely, families giving higher importance to the pattern of conformity orientation communication discourage their children from talking about their feelings and ideas and give importance to the primacy of the parents' opinions and ideas. Families with alcohol addicted parents and/or family elders usually adopt the second type of communication pattern and this communication pattern very often proves to be a stumbling block to the children's growth of self-esteem and self-worth. According to Keaten *et al*[47] in those families children do not try to be free in sharing their views, opinions, feeling and perceptions because of the apprehension of punishment or ignorance from the side of their parents and elders.

Prest and Storm[48] suggested that persistence of alcoholism hampers the ability and skills of the members to express, modulate the emotions and understand the emotional needs of members. As a result of that, these people imbibe compulsive behavioural patterns for coping with the stress of not having the open atmosphere to talk about own feelings and views. These families are at higher risk of experiencing very malevolent form of family conflicts frequently and those conflicts eventually increase the risk of substance misuse. This way a 'vicious cycle' of family conflict and recurrence/maintenance alcohol addiction keeps on prevailing in those families. These families are found to be marred by the problematic issues like unresolved conflicts, denial, breaking down of open communication and mutual caringness among members, and presence of these negative things further trigger the alcohol abuse.

Alcoholism & Parenting/Caregiving to Children

In families where alcohol or other drugs are being abused by one or more member, the general behavioural and communicational pattern of those families is found to be grossly unpredictable and unclear. In those families, family life is found to be very much strained, chaotic and unpredictable. Family structure and rules may appear as either nonexistent or inconsistent. Children of these families very often feel confused and insecure. They love their parents and worry about them, and yet feel angry and hurt that their parents do not love them enough to stop using. Diana Baumrind[49] conceptualized that behavioural characteristics of individuals' are deeply associated with parenting styles. As per Baumrind,[49] children of authoritative parents are likely to have the most desirable behavioural characteristics. These children are found to have good interpersonal skills, higher abilities to establish cooperative relationship with others, high self-controlling abilities, independent, energetic and achievement oriented. Children with low self- esteem and self -control have higher risk to develop addiction in their later life.[50,51] Past studies on the consequences of parental alcoholism (especially fathers) on children suggested that these children are at risk of developing several psychological and behavioural problems like attention and concentration difficulties, impulsive acts, and acts resembling conduct problems during their childhood, and further ramifications in their behavioural regimen are seen in the forms of developing antisocial traits during their adolescence and adulthood.[52-56] Parents with alcohol addiction exhibit marked inadequacies in the forms of 'highly critical to children', 'hostile and punitive to children for trivial reasons', 'lack of emotional involvement in family affairs or with children', 'adoption of erroneous behavioural controlling mechanism' and 'poor guidance to children'.[57, 58]

Alcoholism and Social Relationship & Social Image of the Family

In healthy families, children automatically learn the fact that they are in a safe and supportive environment as well as they are under good supervision and care. This perception eventually generates a sense of confidence in their mind upon the various facets and individuals of their family systems. Their subjective feeling of emotional security, physical safety and well-being ultimately plays a pivotal role in developing their personality, positive growth of their physical and emotional health. From this angle it can be stated that, a healthy and safe environment for a child provides the necessary platform for making him a socially accepted and valued individual. Because, healthy family offers the necessary social skills and exposes children with certain critical social experiences that help them to acquire behavioural skills necessary for a socially accepted and valued citizens in their later life.[59] Past empirical research stated that families possessing specific characteristics like 'prevalence of overt conflicts in family', 'inadequate nurturing', 'presence of emotionally cold and uninvolved relationships among members', and 'adoption of unsupportive and neglectful attitude to most of the members' are the harbingers of development of maladaptive and socially defiant individuals. Along with plethora of psychological and emotional difficulties, individuals belonging to these kinds of families are also found to be socially inept and disintegrative.[59] As per the basic tenets of labeling theory, individuals who are being identified and labeled as deviant drinkers would likely to be stigmatized and subject to impaired social interactions.[60] There are two rationales which are put forward by researchers to be highly associated with the stemming of stigma and social distancing of people possessing specific characteristics, problems or features. Those two factors are 'attribution of responsibility' and 'disruption of social interaction'. More than three decades back Albrecht et al[61] tested the theories explaining how common people develop the idea of social distance towards individuals possessing wide range of stigmatized conditions. In that study Albrecht *et al*[61] gave emphasis on two generally stigmatized people: (a) individuals with different forms of disabilities and (b) so called socially deviant people. These researchers found that people tend to express greater social distance from deviants like alcoholics and drug addicts than from the disabled such as paraplegics and the blind. Alcohol addiction not only causes typical individual and family problems, but also affects the occupational and job performances of the addicted people very significantly. Alcoholism causes massive decline in the productivity. Alcohol addicted people frequently apply for sickness leave and that has substantial economic impact on the individual employees and general social security systems of the nation.[62] Alcohol addiction not only hampers the productivity or occupational performances of employed people but it also leads to massive unemployment in the society. Addicted youths neither have the scopes nor can they develop their occupational skills. Because, these people tend to be preoccupied only in addiction-centred behaviour and activities so they don't show interest to other activities of life. Those people do not give much heed to the importance of employment and keep on concentrating on procuring as well as abusing alcohol. The relationship between alcoholism and occupation related problem/unemployment can be bi-directional, *i.e.* chronic heavy consumption and dependence could cause unemployment and loss of work days and productivity could prove to be costly for employed people.[62-64] The social acceptance and recognition of unemployed people with addiction problem is bound to be lower than that of employed non-addicted persons. Therefore, alcoholism is an important predictor of social image and status of people. Problematic pattern of drinking or more specifically dependence to alcoholic beverages may decline the social status and importance of individuals. Because, problematic pattern of drinking has always been recognized as a form of social deviance.

Alcohol Dependence Syndrome & India: Historical Evolution, Socio-Cultural & Socio-Demographic Factors

(a) Historical Evolution & Brief Epidemiology

The history of production and consumption of alcoholic beverages can be traced in the Ancient literatures, scripts and Mythological contents. Though, the use of alcoholic beverages has never been so rampant and universally prevalent in all stratums of the Indian society like West, but at present Indian Society is not far behind from their Western Counterparts. However, alcohol use has always been an issue of great ambivalence in Indian Culture. The evolutionary history of alcohol consumption patterns in India can be categorized into four distinct historical periods, viz. i) Vedic era (ca. 1500–700 BCE), ii) 700 BCE to 1100 CE, iii) The Period of Islamic Regimes (1100–1800 CE) and The Modern Era (1800 to the present). In ancient period consumption of alcoholic beverages was not so common among people belonging to Higher Castes, *e.g.* Brahmin (scholar-priest).[65] But in last few decades the problem of alcoholism is appeared as a major concern to public health in India. The 2003 National Household Survey of Alcohol and Drug Abuse enumerated the point prevalence of alcohol addiction to be 21.4%.[66] In Western Indian State of Goa, Silva *et al* enumerated the prevalence of hazardous consumption of alcohol among adult males to be 21%.[67] These authors observed that hazardous drinking was more prevalent among male industrial workers, and it was associated with an earlier age of onset of drinking, lower education and being Catholic.[67] They had also found that people involved in hazardous drinking were also at risk of developing common mental illnesses.[67] Recently, Kumar *et al* conducted a community based, cross sectional study on 946 subjects aged 10 years and above, in rural Tamil Nadu, India. They found the prevalence of alcohol as 9.4%. Prevalence of alcohol dependence syndrome was more among males (16.8%) as compared to that among females (1.3%). Mean age of starting of problematic ingestion alcohol was found to be 25.3±9.0 years. After multiple logistic regression analysis, these authors observed that middle age (15–44 years) (OR=3.56), male gender (OR=11.23), illiteracy (OR=6.16), lower education levels (OR=2.57) and smoking (OR=17.78) were independently associated with alcohol use. Among those who have had problematic pattern of alcohol intake, 29.2% (26) were possible hazardous drinkers, 33.7%(30) had probable alcohol dependence and 56.2% (50) had experienced harmful effects.[68] In another study, Kim *et al* studied the pattern as well as prevalence of the use of alcohol in urban slums of southern India. These researchers had screened 2811 men for alcohol use by doing a household-level census in an urban slum in Vellore City, Tamil Nadu, and interviewed 220 age- and area-matched pairs of male drinkers and non-drinkers for the purpose of examining factors associated with alcohol use. They observed that among all men, 46.1% had the history of consumption of alcohol and 31.4% had the history of hazardous drinking (19% increased-risk, 7.7% high-risk and 4.7% dependent drinkers). Factors having close association with the problematic use of alcohol were: involvement in manual labour related occupations (OR 2.08); presence of a common mental disorder (OR 1.50) and smoking (OR 2.08); while Muslim religion was found to be protective factor to alcoholism (OR 0.43). Factors causing increased use of alcohol were: being reported as a non-drinker during the census (OR 3.96); presence of a common mental disorder (OR 3.83); smoking (OR 1.78); drinking before legal age of 21 years (OR 2.71); spending more than `100 per day on alcohol (OR 6.17); and mainly drinking Indian-made foreign liquor (OR 5.45)[69].

(b) Socio-cultural & Socio-demographic Factors of Alcohol Dependence in India

Empirical studies had shown categorically that socio-cultural factors like customs, beliefs, religion, laws and moral values are deeply associated with the initiation and perpetuation of alcohol dependence syndrome.[70-72] In addition to those factors, alcohol Dependence has also been found to be influenced by other factors like globalization, market forces, government policies, media promotion and changing values of Indian society. Individualized and family related factors like family history of alcoholism, impulsivity and hyperactivity, lower socioeconomic status, adverse childhood experiences like abuse (*e.g.*, physical, emotional and sexual), neglect(physical or emotional), observing substance abuse in family, family history of criminality, mental illness of household members, parental discord and illicit drug use, possessing poor social skills, academic failures, exposures to drugs, poor quality of parenting, peer group influences, biological and inherent predisposition towards alcohol dependence.[73-77]

CONCLUSION

Alcoholism has emerged as a global menace and perhaps no nation is said to be immune to this menace. It is indeed a stressful task to live with addicted person in a same household. Addicted individual's daily life activities and behaviours tend to hover between two points, *i.e.* procuring and using of addictive substance. Other things and activities, whatever that may be or how important that may be, remain unattractive or least important to them. But the life of their acquaintances tends to be miserable because of their evil habit. Other family members have to put up extra efforts to fill up the vacuum or address the shortcomings which are being created by those addicted people. The task of putting up extra efforts becomes the source of burden and pressure to those people and the entire family system shows the sign of breaking up or destabilization. Normal routines and daily activities of these families are constantly being interrupted by unexpected events and many a time these people do experience ultimate negative things like 'physical violence and hostility', 'emotional, physical or sexual abuse'. In those families marked incompatibility and disparity could be seen between what is being said and what family members sense or perceive. Essential family functions and structures are markedly affected in those families and because of that those families cannot fulfill the needs of their individual members as well as keep the family situation supportive to all members. Researchers and clinicians have made a consensus that ideal intervention of alcoholism should be holistic and it should include families as a therapeutic agent.

REFERENCES

1. E. Glucksman. Alcohol and accidents. *Br Med Bull* **1994**, 50(1), 76-84.
2. N. Giesbrecht, T.K. Greenfield. Public opinions on alcohol policy issues: a comparison of American and Canadian surveys. *Addiction.* **1999**, 94(4), 521-31.
3. J. Orford. Empowering family and friends: a new approach to the secondary prevention of addiction. *Drug Alcohol Rev* **1994**, 13, 417 – 29.
4. J.G. Barber, B.R. Crisp. The 'pressures to change' approach to working with the partners of heavy drinkers. *Addiction* **1995**, 90, 269 – 76.
5. R. Caetano, M.A. Nelson, C. Cunradi. Intimate partner violence, dependence symptoms and social consequences from drinking among White, Black and Hispanic couples in the United States. *Am J Addict* **2001**, 10, 60 – 9.
6. P. Steinglass. A life history model of the alcoholic family. *Fam Process* **1980**, 19(3), 211-26.
7. P. Steinglass, L. Tislenko, D. Reiss. Stability/instability in the alcoholic marriage: The interrelationships between course of alcoholism, family process, and marital outcome. *Fam Process* **1985**, 24(3), 365-76.
8. E.M. Pattison, E. Kaufmann. Family Therapy in the treatment of alcoholism. In: Langsley MR (ed.). Family Therapy and Major Psychopathology. Grune & Stratton, New York, **1981**; 301–24.
9. M. Hindman. Children of alcoholic parents. *Alcohol Health Res World* **1975-76**, 2-6.
10. E. Wallin, J. Gripenberg, S. Andreasson. Too drunk for a beer? A study of overserving in Stockholm. *Addiction* **2002**, 97, 901-07.
11. H.T. Harbin, H.M. Maziar. The families of drug abusers: A literary review. *Fam Process* **1975**, 14, 411-31.

12. M. Klagsbrun, D.I. Davis. Substance abuse and family interaction. *Fam Process* **1977**, 16, 149-73.

13. N.E. Seldin. The family of the addict: A review of the literature. *Int J Addict* **1972**, 7, 97-107.

14. M.D. Stanton. Drugs and the family. *Marriage Fam Rev* **1979**, 2(1), 1-10.

15. M.D. Stanton. Forum: Family therapy for the drug user: Conceptual and practical considerations. *Drug Forum* **1978**, 6, 203-5.

16. M. Bowen. Family Therapy After Twenty Years. 1975. In S. Arieti, (Ed.), American Handbook of Psychiatry, Vol 5, 2nd edn, NY, Basic Books. Repr. In M. Bowen, **1978**.

17. R.J. Ackerman. Adult Children of Alcoholics: The Effects of Background and Treatment on ACOA Symptoms. *Int J Addict* **1991**, 26(11), 1159-72.

18. R.J. Ackerman. Children of Alcoholics. 2nd ed., Simon & Schuster, New York, **1987**.

19. R.J. Ackerman. Let Go and Grow. Health Communications, Deerfield Beach, FL, **1987**.

20. R.J. Ackerman. Perfect Daughters. Health Communications, Deerfield Beach, FL, **1989**.

21. D.H. Olson. Circumplex model of marital and family systems. *J Fam Ther* **2000**, 22(2), 144-67.

22. B.K. Barber, C. Buehler. Family cohesion and enmeshment. Different constructs, different effects. *J Marriage Fam* **1996**, 58, 433–41.

23. E. Kaufman. Family structures of narcotic addicts. *Int J Addict* **1981**, 16(2), 273-82.

24. R. Velleman. Intergenerational effects – a review of environmentally oriented studies concerning the relationship between parental alcohol problems and family disharmony in the genesis of alcohol and other problems. I: the alcohol literature. *Int J Addict* **1992**, 27(3), 253-80.

25. B.J. Bushman, H.M.Cooper. Effects of alcohol on human aggression: An integrative research review. *Psychol Bull* **1990**, 107(3), 341-54.

26. D.H. Coleman, M.A. Straus. Alcohol abuse and family violence. In E. Gottheil, K.A. Druley, T.E., Skoloda, & H.M. Waxman (Eds.) *Alcohol, drug abuse and aggression* (pp.104-124). Springfield IL: C. Thomas, **1983**.

27. E. Kaufman, M.A. Strauss. Substance abuse as a precipitant of wife abuse victimizations. Am *J Drug Alcohol Abuse* **1989**, 15(2), 173-89.

28. H.A. Liddle, G.A. Dakof. Efficacy of family therapy for drug abuse: Promising but not definitive. *J Marital Fam Ther* **1995**, 21(4), 511-43.

29. T.R. Kosten, H.D. Kleber, C. Morgan. Treatment of cocaine abuse with buprenorphine. *Biol Psychiatry* **1989**, 26(6), 637-9.

30. Rossow. Alcohol and homicide: A cross-cultural comparison of the relationship in 14 European countries. *Addiction* **2001**, 96(1), 77-92.

31. S.J. Wolin, L.A. Bennett, D.L. Noonan, *et.al.* Disrupted family rituals: A factor in the intergenerational transmission of alcoholism. *J Stud Alcohol* **1980**, 41(3), 199-214.

32. L.A. Bennett, S.J. Wolin, D. Reiss. Cognitive, behavioral, and emotional problems among school-age children of alcoholic parents. *Am J Psychiatry* **1988**, 145(2), 185-90.

33. M.A. Schuckit, T.L. Smith. The relationships of a family history of alcohol dependence, a low level of response to alcohol and six domains of life functioning to the development of alcohol use disorders. J Stud Alcohol **2000**, 61, 827–35.

34. M.R. Liepman, T.D. Nirenberg, R.H. Doolittle, *et.al.* Family Functioning of Male Alcoholics and Their Female Partners during Periods of Drinking and Abstinence. *Fam Process* **1989**, 28, 239–49.

35. W. Frankenstein, W.M. Hay, P.E. Nathan. Effects of intoxication on alcoholics' marital communication and problem solving. *J Stud Alcohol* **1985**, 46, 1–6.

36. T. Jacob, N. Dunn, K. Leonard. Patterns of alcohol abuse and family stability. *Alcohol Clin Exp Res* **1983**, 7, 382–85.

37. T. Jacob, D. Ritchey, J. Cvitkovic, *et.al.* Communication styles of alcoholic and nonalcoholic families when drinking and not drinking. *J Stud Alcohol* **1981**, 49, 466–82.

38. T. Jacob, G. Krahn. Marital interaction of alcoholic couples: Comparison with depressed and nondistressed couples. *J Consult Clin Psychol* **1988**, 56, 73–9.

39. H. Kuendig, M.L. Plant, M.A. Plant, *et.al.* Beyond drinking: differential effects of demographic and socioeconomic factors on alcohol-related adverse consequences across European countries. *Eur Addict Res* **2008**, 14(3), 150-60.

40. J.W. Bray, G.A. Zarkin, C. Ringwalt, *et.al.* The relationship between marijuana initiation and dropping out of high school. *Health Econ* **2000**, 9(1), 9–18.

41. S. Minuchin. Families and Family Therapy. Harvard University Press: Cambridge, **1974**.
42. M.C. Haverfield, J.A. Theiss, J. Leustek. Characteristics of Communication in Families of Alcoholics. *J Fam Commun* **2016**, 16(2), 111-27.
43. D.C. Jones, R. Houts. Parental drinking, parent–child communication, and social skills in young adults. *J Stud Alcohol* **1992**, 53, 48–56.
44. P. Johnson. Dimensions of functioning in alcoholic and nonalcoholic families. *J Ment Health Couns* **2001**, 23, 127–36.
45. C. Black. It will never happen to me. Denver, CO: MAC Printing and Publications Division, **1982**.
46. L.D. Ritchie, M.A. Fitzpatrick. Family communication patterns: Measuring intrapersonal perceptions of interpersonal relationships. *Communic Res* **1990**, 17, 523–44.
47. J.A. Keaten, L. Kelly, D.L. Palmer. The role of emotional intelligence in explicating the impact of family communication patterns on reticence. Paper presented at the annual convention of the National Communication Association, Chicago, 2004. As cited in: S Rangarajan, L Kelly. Family communication patterns, family environment, and the impact of parental alcoholism on offspring self-esteem. *J Soc Pers Relat* **2006**, 23(4), 655–71.
48. L. Prest, C. Storm. The codependent relationships of compulsive eaters and drinkers: Drawing Parallels. *Am J Fam Ther* **1988**, 16, 339-49.
49. D. Baumrind. The influence of parenting style on adolescent competence and substance use. *J Early Adolesc* **1991**, 11(1), 56-95.
50. A.F. Brennan, S. Walfish, P. Aubuchon. Alcohol use and abuse in college students. II. Social/environmental correlates, methodological issues, and implications for intervention. *Int J Addict* **1986**,21(4-5), 475-93.
51. A.F. Brennan, S. Walfish, P. AuBuchon. Alcohol use and abuse in college students. I. A review of individual and personality correlates. *Int J Addict* **1986**, 21(4-5), 449-74.
52. L. Chassin, F. Rogosch, M. Barrera. Substance use and symptomatology among adolescent children of alcoholics. *J Abnorm Psychol* **1991**, 100, 449–63.
53. S. Johnson, K.E. Leonard, T. Jacob. Drinking, drinking styles, and drug use in children of alcoholics, depressives, and controls. *J Stud Alcohol* **1989**, 50, 427–31.
54. M.O. West, R.J. Prinz. Parental alcoholism and childhood psychopathology. *Psychol Bull* **1987**, 102, 204–18.
55. R.A. Zucker. Developmental aspects of drinking through the young adult years. In: H.T. Blane, M.E. Chafetz, editors. Youth, alcohol, and social policy. Plenum Press; New York: **1979**.

56. R.A. Zucker, E.S.L. Gomberg. Etiology of alcoholism reconsidered: The case for a biopsychosocial process. *Am Psychol* **1986**, 41, 783–93.
57. R.D. Eiden, K.E. Leonard, R.H. Hoyle, *et.al.* A transactional model of parent–infant interactions in alcoholic families. *Psychol Addict Behav* **2004**, 18, 350–61.
58. L.K. Kachadourian, R.D. Eiden, K.E. Leonard. Paternal alcoholism, negative parenting, and the mediating role of marital satisfaction. *Addict Behav* **2009**, 34(11), 918–27.
59. R.L.Repetti, S. Taylor, T.E. Seeman. Risky families: Family social environments and the mental and physical health of offspring. *Psychol Bull* **2002**, 128(2), 330–66.
60. D.M.Tootle. Social acceptance of the recovering alcoholic in the workplace: A research note. *J Drug Issues* **1987**, 17(3), 273-79.
61. G.L. Albrecht, V.G. Walker, J.A. Levy. Social distance from the stigmatized: A test of two theories. *Soc Sci Med* **1982**, 16(14), 1319-27.
62. H. Klingemann, G. Gmel. Mapping the Social Consequences of Alcohol Consumption. Dordrecht, Netherlands: Kluwer Academic Publishers, **2001**.
63. J. Mullahy, J.L. Sindelar. Alcoholism, work, and income. *J Labor Econ* **1993**, 11, 494-520.
64. J. Mullahy, J.L. Sindelar. Health, income, and risk aversion: Assessing some welfare costs of alcoholism and poor health. *J Human Resources* **1995**, 30, 439-60.
65. H.K. Sharma, B.M. Tripathi, P.J. Pelto. The evolution of alcohol use in India. *AIDS Behav* **2010**, 14, 8-17.
66. The National Household Survey of Alcohol and Drug Abuse. New Delhi, Clinical Epidemiological Unit, All India Institute of Medical Sciences, **2004**.
67. M.C. Silva, G. Gaunekar, V. Patel, *et.al.* The prevalence and correlates of hazardous drinking in industrial workers: A study from Goa, India. *Alcohol Alcohol* **2003**, 38, 79–83.
68. S. Ganesh Kumar, K.C. Premarajan, L. Subitha, *et.al.* Prevalence and pattern of alcohol consumption using Alcohol Use Disorders Identification Test (AUDIT) in rural Tamil Nadu, India. *J Clin Diagn Res* **2013**, 7(8), 1637–9.
69. S. Kim, S. Rifkin, S.M. John, *et.al.* Nature, prevalence and risk factors of alcohol use in an urban slum of Southern India. *Natl Med J India* **2013**, 26(4), 203-9.
70. B.T. Vignesh, A.K. Singh, S.K. Mohan, *et.al.* Association between Socio-Demographics and Alcohol Dependence among Individuals Living in an Indian Setting. *Glob J Health Sci* **2014**, 6(3), 16–26.

71. Pillai, M.B. Nayak, T.K. Greenfield, *et.al.* Patterns of alcohol use, their correlates, and impact in male drinkers: a population-based survey from Goa, India. *Soc Psychiatry Psychiatr Epidemiol* **2013**, 48(2), 275–82.
72. A.P. Sarkar, S. Sen, S. Mondal, *et.al.* A study on socio-demographic characteristics of alcoholics attending the de-addiction center at Burdwan medical college and hospital in West Bengal. *Indian J Public Health* **2013**, 57(1), 33-5.
73. S.A. Malhotra. Comparison of beliefs of Indian alcohol dependent patients and their close family members on their reasons for relapse. *Addiction* **1999**, 94(3), 709-13.
74. P. Prabhu, R. Srinivas, K. Vishwanathan. Factors influencing alcohol and tobacco addiction among patients attending a de-addiction Centre, South India. *J Int Soc Prev Community Dent* **2014**, 4(2), 103–7.
75. R. Lal. Substance Use Disorders: A Manual for physicians. New Delhi: National Drug Dependence Treatment Center, All India Institute of Medical Sciences, **2005**.
76. S.K. Das, V. Balakrishnan, D.M. Vasudevan. Alcohol: Its health and social impact in India. *Med Soc* **2006**, 19(2), 94-9.
77. K.J. Neufeld, D.H. Peters, M. Rani, *et.al.* Regular use of alcohol and tobacco in India and its association with age, gender, and poverty. *Drug Alcohol Depen* **2005**, 77(3), 283-91.

Editors' Note

An alcoholic person is not only an economic burden on the family but also a source of continuous psychological strain which leads to disruption in mutual relationships with family and friends. The essential functioning of family and family structures as well are markedly affected in alcoholics' families. Disturbances in family due to alcoholics affects whole family (including kids) as such families cannot fulfill the needs of their individual members as well as unable to keep the family situation supportive to all members. Remedy to such a problem lies in combining together psychotherapies, medical care and de-addiction efforts with the consideration and holistic involvement of family and friends.

❑❑❑

3

The Effects of Alcoholism on the Brain

Ram Singh*, Geetanjali and Deepak Mishra***

ABSTRACT

Alcohol abuse and alcoholism is an age old practice and is the reflection of socio-cultural factors of society. Drinking alcohol is as much a part of daily life as having food and even sometime people prefer to have alcohol than food. People who have been drinking excess amounts of alcohol for longer periods of time are exposing themselves to the risk of developing serious and persistent changes in various organs including the brain. The effect of alcohol on the brain may be direct or indirect depending upon general health status of the person. The studies have suggested that the brain functions are affected due to interaction of alcohol with multiple neurotransmitter systems. This chapter will discuss the effect of alcohol in the brain.

Keywords: Alcohol, Ethanol, Brain, Acetaldehyde, CNS

INTRODUCTION

Alcohol, in chemistry, is a group of organic compound in which a saturated carbon atom is attached to the hydroxyl (-OH) functional group. This is

* Department of Applied Chemistry, Delhi Technological University, Delhi-110 042, India.

** Department of Chemistry, Kirori Mal College, University of Delhi, Delhi-110 007, India.

represented as R-OH. All alcohols are not suitable for drinking purposes. Only the ethyl alcohol (CH_3CH_2OH; ethanol) has been found to be suitable for drinking and hence is being used in the production of alcoholic beverages. This is the most widely consumed chemical worldwide. In general, people use the term 'alcohol' informally for ethanol in all drinking purposes. Drinking alcohol is an age old practice and is the reflection of socio-cultural factors of society.[1] All the rural and urban societies have been using the fermented alcoholic beverages till the modern concept of alcoholic drinks get introduced. People have a misconception about the alcohol drinking that this releases their tension and makes them happy. But the fact is, ethanol is a psychoactive substance and possess more adverse effect than positive effect. The adverse effect includes various disorders and diseases, a social and economic burden in societies. However, these effects are highly dependent on the volume and quality of alcohol consumed and the pattern of drinking adopted.[1]

The consumption of alcohol is worldwide irrespective of caste, creed, religion and gender in the forms like beer, wine, spirits or other alcoholic beverages.[1] According to the World Health Organization (WHO) data, individuals above 15 years of age drink on an average 6.2 liters of pure alcohol per year worldwide as per 2014 report.[2] The report says that the highest consumption levels are found in the developed world which includes the WHO European Region (EUR) and the WHO Region of the Americas (AMR). The WHO Western Pacific Region (WPR) and the WHO African Region (AFR) come under the category of intermediate levels of consumption. The WHO South-East Asia Region (SEAR) and the WHO Eastern Mediterranean Region are among the lowest consumption levels.[2] The alcohol consumption is directly linked with the economic condition of the country. The higher economic wealth of a country showed more alcohol consumption.

According to Dr. Ala Alwan, World Health Organization, "Alcohol problems are of global scale, but they can be reduced and prevented. Amidst rapid globalization, drinking patterns are worsening, often in places with the fewest resources to combat them. Global leadership is needed for this global problem." The alcohol consumption ranks among the top five risk factors for disease, disability, and death throughout the world.[3] This problem is associated with numerous social consequences, such as crimes, violence, unemployment and absenteeism. The alcohol drinking habit increases the health-care and societal costs and also contributes significantly to the disparities in health between and within the countries.

Ethanol is classified as depressant.[4] The damaging effects of this in CNS are possible either from its direct toxic effect or from an indirect effect involving its metabolites or reactive oxygen species (ROS) generation. The ethanol drinking slows down the vital functions and results in unsteady movement, an inability to react quickly, slurred speech and disturbed precipitations. The amount of ethanol consumed determines the type of effect. Its overdose causes a more severe depressant effect such as an inability to feel pain, unconsciousness, worse, coma or even death. Ethanol can travel anywhere in our body as they contain both hydrocarbon chain and hydroxyl group and hence the hydrophobic part allows them to move into fat while the hydroxyl group (hydrophilic part) allows moving into water.[4]

Alcohols are absorbed into the bloodstream *via* small blood vessels in the walls of the stomach and small intestine. An approximately 20% of alcohol is absorbed through the stomach while the rest 80% is absorbed through the small intestine. Within few minutes of drinking of alcohol, it travels up to the brain from the stomach, where it produces it effects and slow down the function of nerve cells. When the amount of alcohol in the blood exceeds a certain limit, the respiratory system slows down and cause coma. In addition, this also affects many other vital organ systems. Cirrhosis of the liver is another example. This is the ninth leading cause of death in the world. Also, alcohol abuse significantly increases the risk of developing certain types of cancer. This has also been observed in alcohol binge-drinking rats that during alcohol exposure, the proliferation of neural stem cells and the survival of neurons produced from the stem cells are decreased.[5] The chronic exposure to human also leads to ample reductions in the prefrontal cortex and cerebellum part of the brain.[6] The orbitofrontal cortex portion of the prefrontal cortex is involved in high-level cognitive and executive functions. The deficits in these brain areas may impact the cognitive and executive functions.[7] This chapter gives comprehensive coverage of mechanisms by which alcohol consumption may influence behaviour through its interaction with multiple neurotransmitter systems.

OXIDATION OF ETHANOL IN THE BRAIN

The chronic and excessive consumption of ethanol cause damage to brain[8] like it does with other organs of the body such as heart, liver, and the bile.[9-12]. The quantum of damage and neuro-behavioral effect changes from person to person depending upon the quantity and time period of ethanol consumption. The effect also depends on age, gender, family history and level of education of the person. A number of studies for the effects of ethanol consumption on brain have been done and postulated to be mediated through acetaldehyde (CH_3CHO), the first metabolite of ethanol.[13-18]

Acetaldehyde plays a crucial role in the alcoholic people and is responsible for the behavioural, neurochemical and neurotoxic actions.[13,19-21] However, this hypothesis has several doubts and is still under investigation. The hypothesis failed to answer the following doubts:

(*i*) The level of acetaldehyde in most of the people is nearly undetectable in their blood stream after consumption of ethanol.[22]

(*ii*) Substantial amount of acetaldehyde is required to cross the blood–brain barrier through the substantial blood levels in the brain.[23-26] The amount of acetaldehyde keeps low due to the fact that the enzyme aldehyde dehydrogenase (ALDH) present in blood-brain barrier converts acetaldehyde to acetate.[27,28]

(*iii*) The oxidation of ethanol by alcohol dehydrogenase (ADH) was inhibited by pyrazole, still intoxication resulted created doubt about the role of only acetaldehyde.[29, 30]

Several groups have reported the oxidation of ethanol in the brain.[13,25,31-34] (Figure 1). The three enzymes that are involved in the metabolism of ethanol to acetaldehyde in the brain are *Catalase*, *Cytochrome P450* and *Alcohol dehydrogenase* (ADH).[35]

Catalase [EC 1.11.1.6] catalyzes the breakdown of hydrogen peroxide (H_2O_2) to oxygen (O_2) and water (H_2O). This enzyme metabolizes ethanol (CH_3CH_2OH) and converts it to acetaldehyde (CH_3CHO) in the brain with the help of hydrogen peroxide.[33,34,36]

Cytochrome P4502E1 (CYP2E1 [EC 1.14.13.n7]) enzymes are capable of oxidizing ethanol efficiently in other tissues that are found in the brain.[37-39] The model studies in rats and mice had shown the involvement of cytochrome P450 in metabolism of ethanol to acetaldehyde in the brain.[35]

Alcohol dehydrogenases (ADH; [EC 1.1.1.1]) are the enzymes involved in the inter-conversion between alcohols and aldehydes or ketones. Several groups had reported that only the subtypes ADH1, ADH3, and ADH4 are present in the brain.[40-43] Martinez and colleagues found mRNA for ADH1 and ADH4 in rat brain cells.[44]

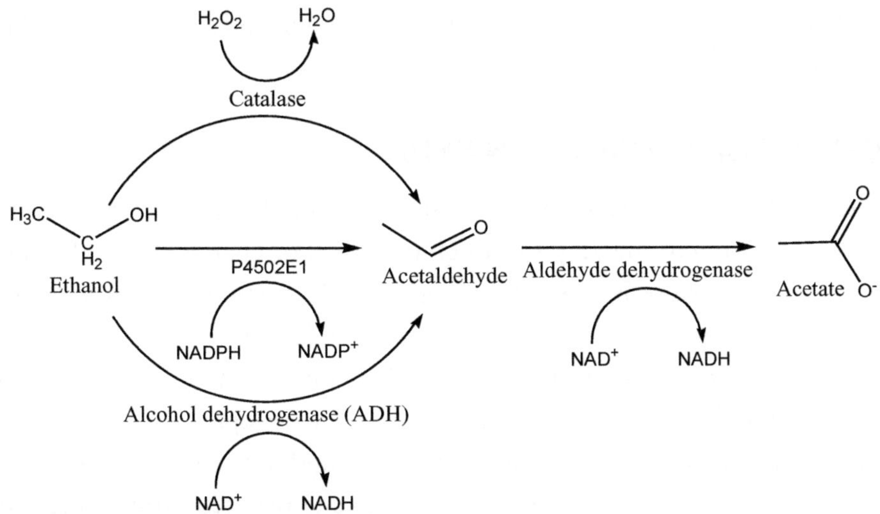

Fig. 1: Possible pathways of ethanol metabolism in brain

The quantity of acetaldehyde in the brain at a particular period is dependent on the comparative rate of removal and formation of acetaldehyde. This is because substantial amounts of acetaldehyde are oxidized to acetate in the systems. Hence, to study the exact damage done by the acetaldehyde in the brain need to overcome these limitations.[35]

EFFECT OF ETHANOL ON ASTROCYTES IN THE CNS

Astrocytes are specialized glial cells and continuously cover the entire central nervous system (CNS).[45] The glial cells represent the majority cell population in the CNS. Their population is 10 to 50 times more than the neurons in the CNS. They surround neurons and hold them in place and also perform a number of other functions in the brain.[46-49]

Ethanol has several targets in astrocytes and induces astroglial activation, associated with up-regulation of several pro-inflammatory cytokines that is responsible for cell apoptosis neuroinflammation and neurodegeneration.[50,51] The developing brain also gets affected by ethanol drinking. The glycoproteins help in the nervous system development and ethanol affects the synthesis, intracellular transport, distribution, and secretin of N-glycoproteins in astrocytes and neurons leading to hindrance in brain development.[52] Ethanol has an extensive array of actions on astrocytes, transforming them into activated, potentially injurious cells with negative consequences for neuronal function and survival and to brain function.[50,51]

EFFECT OF ETHANOL ON SYNAPSES

The human brain is made up of billion of neurons. These neurons help in the communication of messages through electrical or chemical signal to other neurons. A synapse is a structure that helps the neurons (or nerve cells) to pass the messages.[53] The continuous intake of ethanol affects the synaptic structure.[54] The synaptic plasticity and memory function are controlled by N-methyl-D-aspartate receptor (NMDA receptor or NMDAR).[55] The NMDA receptor is a glutamate receptor and ion channel protein found in nerve cells.[56] Glutamate is important excitatory neurotransmitters that increases the activity of signal receiving neurons and play a major role in controlling the brain function. It exerts its effects on cell in part through three types of receptors that, when activated, allow the flow of positively charged ions into the cell. This receptor is a major target of ethanol in the brain and is associated with ethanol tolerance, dependence, withdrawal, craving, and relapse.[57-59] The low level of ethanol concentration inhibits the excitary activity of the NMDA receptor, which contributes towards the abnormalities like learning disabilities, neuronal losses and cognitive deficits.

The subunits of the NMDA receptor form a cation channel. The permeability for cations of sodium (Na^+), potassium (K^+) and calcium (Ca^{2+}) increases due to the activation of the receptor leading to the depolarization of the neuronal membrane.[60,61] The flow through the channel gets reduced due to action of ethanol on this receptor.[62] This modification in the flow changes the synaptic function by inhibiting the release of neurotransmitters including dopamine, norepinephrine, and acetylcholine[63] and hence affects learning and memory.[64,65] The continuous ethanol consumption leads to an adaptive up-regulation of NMDA receptor function in animal brains.[61] The withdrawal produces alcohol withdrawal syndrome including a psychotic condition involving tremors, hallucinations, anxiety, and disorientation.[66]

The exact mechanism and direct action for changes in the functionality of this receptor by ethanol remains unclear.[67] The possible mechanism of action is to interfere with the phosphorylation and compartmentalization of this receptor.[68,69] The inhibition of the NMDA receptors by ethanol is mainly restricted in the subset of neurons.[70] This is because the different sub-units of the receptors have different sensitivity to ethanol.[71]

Ethanol also interacts with another membrane receptor, γ-aminobutyric acid (4-aminobutyric acid, GABA). GABA occurs in 30-40% of all synapses and is the principal inhibitory neurotransmitter present in the brain. The GABA system plays an important role in the behavioral and pharmacological effects of ethanol. There are three types of GABA receptors, $GABA_A$, $GABA_B$ and $GABA_C$. $GABA_A$ and $GABA_C$ receptors are ligand-gated whereas $GABA_B$ receptors are G protein-coupled receptors.[72]

$GABA_A$ receptor protein complex is composed of five subunits, which forms a channel across the neuronal membrane for chloride ions. In addition to the main activator of this receptor, the GABA, there are many other substances that interact with this complex. These substances bind to different parts of the receptor, either in the extracellular region or in the channel domain, leading to the modulation in the anion channel activity.[72,73] Ethanol does not affect all the subunits of all types of GABA. The sensitivity of ethanol is only restricted to certain subtypes of some subunits.[74,75] The chronic consumption leads to the decreased sensitivity of $GABA_A$ receptor-mediated responses.[76] Ethanol does not directly bind to the site rather this act allosterically and potentiates the action of GABA.[77,78] The allosteric effect is the binding of a molecule to the site other than the active site of an enzyme. This type of binding changes the shape of active site and modulates the enzyme activity. The modulation of receptor leads to the stimulation of the flow of chloride ion.[77,78] Few studies have also suggested that the modulation of the $GABA_A$ receptor is not only done by the direct allosteric effect of ethanol rather phosphorylation/dephosphorylation mechanisms are also important.[74] The ethanol dependence and withdrawal are also responsible for the various polymorphisms in the $GABA_A$ gene[79] and there is a possibility of significant functional consequences.[80]

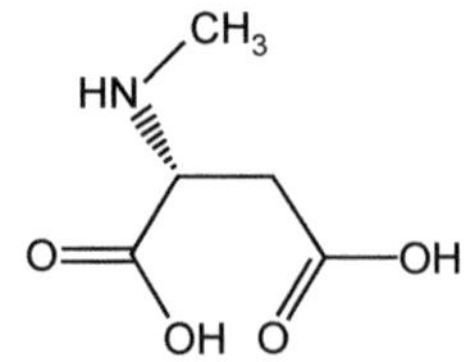

(2R)-2-(methylamino) succinic acid (NMDA)

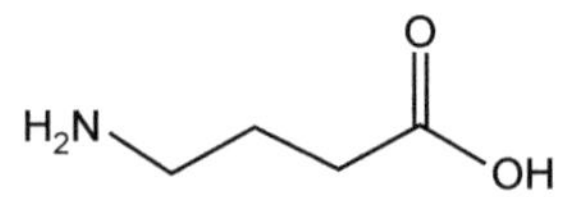

4-Aminobutyric acid (GABA)

Another GABA receptor, $GABA_B$ is very useful in regulating membrane excitability and synaptic transmission in the brain.[81] This receptor is a G protein-coupled receptor and hence signals mainly through activation of G proteins using potassium and calcium channels.[82] Ethanol enhances the $GABA_B$ induced synaptic responses. The activation of this receptor leads to an inhibition of the cation channels. This results in a hyperpolarization of the membrane and a consequent decrease in neuronal excitability[83] and altered mental and motor performance in an acute intoxication phase.[84]

EFFECT OF ETHANOL ON OTHER NEUROTRANSMITTERS

Ethanol being small molecule interacts with many neurotransmitter systems in the brain.[85] The mesocorticolimbic dopamine (DA) system plays an important roles in motivation, reward, memory, learning, and movement.[86,87] Ethanol acutely activates this system and, upon consumption for longer period of life span results in functional changes to the brain reward system.[88,89] The studies have suggested that the ethanol has both positive and negative reinforcing effects on this system.[90] The *in vivo* and *in vitro* studies have shown that the ethanol caused dose-dependent excitation of dopaminergic ventral tegmental area (VTA) neurons.[91] The polymorphic variations in many dopaminergic system genes have been observed in alcoholics.[92] Also, increase in polymorphism observed in the dopamine transporter gene in alcoholics with severe alcohol withdrawal symptoms.[93]

Serotonin (5-hydroxytryptamine or 5-HT) is a monoamine neurotransmitter and involved in different aspects of brain functions like addiction, ingestive behaviour etc.[94] The ethanol consumption increases the function of the 5-HT3 and 5-HT1A receptors[95] and also increases the extracellular serotonin levels in the nucleus accumbens.[96] The ethanol addictions were also associated with a particular polymorphism of the serotonin transporter.[97]

EFFECT OF ETHANOL ON MEMORY

Some of the brain functions like memory, consciousness, alertness, and learning are controlled by multiple neurotransmitter and neuromodulatory systems. In the case of memory, researchers have postulated that information is stored in the brain as a change in the level of communication across synapses produced by an external event such as a sight or sound.[98] A phenomenon called long-term potentiation (LTP) appears to be fundamental for memory formation.[98] LTP is a sudden but lasting increase in the overall level of excitatory neurotransmission in the hippocampus. In general, LTP seems to require activation of glutamate receptors and inhibition of GABAA receptors.

Some studies have shown that short-term alcohol exposure inhibits glutamate receptor function[99] and stimulates GABAA receptor function in the hippocampus.[100] Therefore, it appears that alcohol might inhibit LTP. Thus, if LTP does play a role in memory storage processes, alcohol's general inhibitory effect on memory could be related in part to its effects on glutamate and GABA systems.[101,102]

EFFECT OF ETHANOL ON BRAIN DEVELOPMENT

The effects of alcohol on the brain development are diverse and mediated by many internal and external factors. The brain development are mostly get affected by alcohol in teenagers because their brains are more sensitive than adults brain. There are two area of the brain that are particularly sensitive to alcohol during brain development *i.e.* hippocampus and prefrontal lobe. The hippocampus is the part of the limbic system, and is intimately involved in motivation and emotion, it also plays a central role in the formation of memories and learning.[103,104] It is located deep under the brain surface and is connected with the outer layer of the brain called neocortex. Studies of adolescent shows that there is 10% reduction in the size of hippocampus by heavy and extended alcohol use and is poisonous to the nerve cell of hippocampus causing them to be damaged or destroyed.[105]

EFFECT OF ETHANOL ON BEHAVIOUR

The behaviour of any person depends upon the individual blood alcohol concentration (BAC) and how frequent the person maintains the BAC level. However, the definition of behavior is itself very diverse and is combination of many features. The low BAC level usually has a stimulating effect whereas high concentration leads to depressant effect.[106] The behavior of alcoholics also depends upon the individual tolerance to acute intoxication.[106] There is a general believe that the alcohol consumption leads to intolerance, aggression with violent crimes.[107,108] The alcoholics get frustrated very easily and lacks goal oriented behavior. This prompted them to further increase the intake amount of alcohol which only worsens their condition with time.

SUMMARY

Ethanol is one of the most commonly used and abused chemical compound on this earth since beginning of humankind. Drinking ethanol is a devastating chronic and progressive disorder that makes a person ethanol tolerant and dependent. This is one of the current threats to the health and safety of people globally. This is a known sedative and depressant acting on a wide range of targets including several neurotransmitter receptors and ion channels in the central nervous system. The studies have suggested that the adverse effect of ethanol consumption is mainly due to its first metabolite, acetaldehyde. Acetaldehyde plays a crucial role in the alcoholic people and is responsible for the behavioural, neurochemical and neurotoxic actions. Also, ethanol has several targets in astrocytes and responsible for cell apoptosis neuroinflammation and neurodegeneration. The interaction of ethanol with multiple neurotransmitter system is associated with ethanol tolerance, dependence, withdrawal symptoms, relapses etc. The society whether rural or urban, needs to take proper care of coming generations to avoid them to get into the trap of alcoholism.

ACKNOWLEDGMENTS

The authors are thankful to Council of Scientific & Industrial Research (*CSIR*), India, for financial support.

REFERENCES

1. P. McGovern. Uncorking the past: The quest for wine, beer, and other alcoholic beverages, Berkley (CA): University of California Press, **2009**.
2. Global status report on alcohol and health, World Health Organization (WHO), **2014**.
3. http://www.who.int/nmh/publications/fact_sheet_alcohol_en.pdf (retrieved on March 13, **2016**).
4. G. Hanson, P. Venturelli, A. Fleckenstein. Drugs and Society, Jones & Bartlett Publishers, pp. 201, **2011.**
5. K. Nixon, F.T. Crews. Binge ethanol exposure decreases neurogenesis in adult rat hippocampus. *J. Neurochem*. **2002**, 83, 1087-1093.

6. E.V. Sullivan, A. Pfefferbaum. Neurocircuitry in alcoholism: a substrate of disruption and repair. *Psychopharmacol. (Berl).* **2005**, 180, 583-594.
7. J.D. Jentsch, J.R. Taylor. Impulsivity resulting from frontostriatal dysfunction in drug abuse: implications for the control of behavior by reward-related stimuli. *Psychopharmacol. (Berl).* **1999**, 146, 373-390.
8. C. Montoliu, M. Sancho-Tello, I. Azorin, M. Burgal, S. Valler, J. Renan, C. Guerri. Ethanol increases cytochrome P4502E1 and induced oxidative stress in astmcytes. *J. Neurochem.* **1995**, 65, 2561-2570.
9. K.T. Knecht, B.U. Bradford, R.P. Mason, R.G. Thurman. *In vivo* formation of a free radical metabolite of ethanol. *Mol. Pharmacol.* **1990**, 38, 26-30.
10. K.T. Knecht, Y. Adachi, B.U. Bradford, Y. Iimaro, M. Kadiiska, X.Q. Hui, R.G. Thurman. Free Radical adducts in the bile of rats treated chronically with intragastric alcohol. Inhibition by destruction of Kupffer cells. *Mol. Pharmacol.* **1995**, 47, 1028-1034.
11. L.A. Reinke, E.K. Lai, L.M. DuBose, P.B. McCay. Reactive free radical generation *in vivo* heart and liver of ethanol-fed rats: Correlations with radical formation in vitro. *Proc. Natl. Acad. Sci. USA* **1987**, 84, 9223-9227.
12. L.A. Reinke, Y. Katoki, P.B. McCay, E.G. Janzen. Spin-trapping studies of hepatic free radicals formed following the acute administration of ethanol to rats: *In vivo* detection of 1-hydroxylradicals with PBN. *Free Rad. Biol. Med.* **1991**, 11, 31-39.
13. W.A. Hunt. Role of acetaldehyde in the actions of ethanol on the brain: A review. *Alcohol.* **1996**, 13, 147-151.
14. T. Hashimoto, T. Ueha, T. Kuriyama, M. Katsura, K. Kuriyama. Acetaldehyde-induced alterations in metabolism of monoamines in mouse brain. *Alcohol Alcohol.* **1989**, 24, 91–99.
15. S.M. Zimatkin, R. Deitrich. Ethanol metabolism in the brain. *Addiction Biol.* **1997**, 2, 387–399.
16. P.V. Thadani, E.B. Truitt Jr. Effect of acute ethanol or acetaldehyde administration on the uptake, release, metabolism and turnover of norepinephrine in rat brain. *Biochem. Pharmacol.* **1977**, 26, 1147–1150.
17. M.A. Collins, N.S. Ung-Chhun, K. Raikoff. Stable acetaldehyde adducts with brain proteins. *Alcohol Alcohol.* **1988**, 23, 23-31.
18. L. Heap, R.J. Ward, C. Abiaka, D. Dexter, M. Lawlor, O. Pratt, A. Thomson, K. Shaw, T.J. Peters. The influence of brain acetaldehyde on oxidative status, dopamine metabolism and visual discrimination task. *Biochem. Pharmacol.* **1995**, 50, 263–270.
19. M.F. Mayo-Smith. Pharmacological management of alcohol withdrawal. A meta-analysis and evidence-based practice guideline. American Society

of Addiction Medicine Working group on pharmacological management of alcohol withdrawal. *JAMA* **1997**, 278, 144-151.

20. J. Brick. Handbook of the medical consequences of alcohol and drug abuse. Routledge. **2012**.
21. P.J. Brooks, D. Goldman, T.K. Li. Alleles of alcohol and acetaldehyde metabolism genes modulate susceptibility to oesophageal cancer from alcohol consumption. *Hum. Genomics*, **2009**, 3, 103-105.
22. H.W. Sippel, C.J. Eriksson. The acetaldehyde content in rat brain during ethanol oxidation. In: K.O. Lindros, C.J. Eriksson, eds. The Role of Acetaldehyde in the Actions of Ethanol, Satellite Symposium 6th International Congress Pharmacology. Helsinki, Finland: The Finnish Foundation for Alcohol Studies, **1975**, 149–157.
23. B. Tabakoff, R.A. Anderson, R.F. Ritzmann. Brain acetaldehyde after ethanol administration. *Biochem. Pharmacol.* **1976**, 25, 1305–1309.
24. J.Y. Westcott, H. Weiner, J. Schultz, R.D. Myers. In vivo acetaldehyde in the brain of the rat treated with ethanol. *Biochem. Pharmacol.* **1980**, 29, 411–417.
25. H.W. Sippel. The acetaldehyde content in rat brain during ethanol metabolism. *J. Neurochem.* **1974**, 23, 451–452.
26. S.M. Zimatkin, P.S. Pronko. Levels of ethanol and acetaldehyde and morphological disturbances in brain following administration of alcohol and ALDH inhibitors. In: B. Jacob, W. Bonte, eds. International Association of Forensic Science. Verlag, Berlin, 1-4, **1995**.
27. D.R. Petersen. Aldehyde dehydrogenase and aldehyde reductase in isolated bovine brain microvessels. *Alcohol* **1985**, 2, 79–83.
28. L. Tampier, S. Cariz, M.E. Quintanilla. Metabolism of acetaldehyde by rat isolated aortic rings: Does endothelial tissue contribute to its extrahepatic metabolism? *Alcohol* **1993**, 10, 203–206.
29. E.A. Rekka, P.N. Kourounakis. Chemistry and molecular aspects of drug design and action, CRC Press, pp. 49, **2008**.
30. D.B. Goldstein, R. Zaechelein. Time course of functional tolerance produced in mice by inhalation of ethanol. *J. Pharmacol. Exp. Ther.* **1983**, 227, 150-153.
31. J. Wanga, H. Du, L. Jiang, X. Ma, R.A. de Graaf, K.L. Behar, G.F. Mason. Oxidation of ethanol in the rat brain and effects associated with chronic ethanol exposure. *Proc. Nat. Acad. Sci. USA* **2013**, 110, 14444–14449.
32. C.M. Aragon, F. Rogan, Z. Amit. Ethanol metabolism in rat brain homogenates by a catalase-H_2O_2 system. *Biochem. Pharmacol.* **1992**, 44, 93-98.

33. S.M. Zimatkin, A.L. Buben. Ethanol oxidation in the living brain. *Alcohol Alcohol.* **2007**, 42, 529-532.

34. G. Cohen, P.M. Sinet, R. Heikkila. Ethanol oxidation by rat brain *in vivo*. *Alcohol. Clin. Exp. Res.* **1980**, 4, 366–370.

35. R. Deitrich, S. Zimatkin, S. Pronko. Oxidation of ethanol in the brain and its consequences. *Alcohol Res. Health.* **2006**, 29, 266-273.

36. S.M. Zimatkin, A.V. Liopo, R.A. Deitrich. Oxidation of ethanol to acetaldehyde in brain and the possible behavioral consequences. *Adv. Exp. Med. Biol.* **1999**, 463, 231–236.

37. T. Hansson, N. Tindberg, M. Ingelman-Sundberg, C. Kohler. Regional distribution of ethanol-inducible cytochrome P450 IIE1 in the rat central nervous system. *Neurosci.* **1990**, 34, 451–463.

38. M. Warner, J.A. Gustafsson. Effect of ethanol on cytochrome P450 in the rat brain. *Proc. Nat. Acad. Sci. USA* **1994**, 91, 1019–1023.

39. M. Khalighi, M.R. Brzezinski, H. Chen, M.R. Juchau. Inhibition of human prenatal biosynthesis of all-*trans*-retinoic acid by ethanol, ethanol metabolites, and products of lipid peroxidation reactions: A possible role for CYP2E1. *Biochem. Pharmacol.* **1999**, 57, 811–821.

40. T.B. Beisswenger, B. Holmquist, B.L. Vallee. Chi-ADH is the sole alcohol dehydrogenase isozyme of mammalian brains: Implications and inferences. *Proc. Nat. Acad. Sci. USA*. **1985**, 82, 8369– 8373.

41. J.T. Kerr, D.S. Maxwell, D.W. Crabb. Immunocytochemistry of alcohol dehydrogenase in the rat central nervous system. *Alcohol. Clin. Exp. Res.* **1989**, 13, 730–736.

42. R. Buhler, D. Pestalozzi, M. Hess, J.P. Von Wartburg. Immunohistochemical localization of alcohol dehydrogenase in human kidney, endocrine organs and brain. *Pharmacol. Biochem. Behav.* **1983**, 18(Suppl. 1), 55–59.

43. P.R. Giri, M.Linnoila, J.B. O'Neill, D. Goldman. Distribution and possible metabolic role of class III alcohol dehydrogenase in the human brain. *Brain Res.* **1989**, 481, 131–141.

44. S.E. Martinez, J. Vaglenova, J. Sabria, M.C. Martínez, J. Farrés, X. Parés. Distribution of alcohol dehydrogenase mRNA in the rat central nervous system: Consequences for brain ethanol and retinoid metabolism. *Eur. J. Biochem.* **2001**, 268, 5045–5056.

45. M.V. Sofroniew, H.V. Vinters. Astrocytes: biology and pathology. *Acta Neuropathol*. 2010, 119, 7–35.

46. K. Braet, K. Paemeleire, K. D'Herde, M.J. Sanderson, L. Leybaert. Astrocyte endothelial cell calcium signals conveyed by two signalling pathways. *Eur. J. Neurosci.* **2001**, 13, 79-91.

47. A. González, G.M. Salido. Ethanol alters the physiology of neuron-glia communication. *Inter. Rev. Neurobiol.* **2009**, 88, 168-199.

48. B. Grafstein, S. Liu, M.L. Cotrina, S.A. Goldman. Nedergaard M. Meningeal cells can communicate with astrocytes by calcium signaling. *Ann. Neurol.* **2000**, 47, 18-25.

49. P.G. Haydon. Glia: listening and talking to the synapse. *Nature Rev. Neurosci.* **2001**, 2, 185-193.

50. S. Alfonso-Loeches, M. Pascual-Lucas, A.M. Blanco, I. Sanchez-Vera, C. Guerri. Pivotal role of TLR4 Receptors in alcohol-induced neuroinflammation and brain damage. *J. Neurosci.* **2010**, 30, 8285– 8295.

51. L. Šarc, M. Lipnik-Štangelj. Comparison of ethanol and acetaldehyde toxicity in rat astrocytes in primary culture. *Arch. Indust. Hyg. Toxicol.* **2009**, 60, 297-305.

52. A. Braza-Boïls, M. Tomás, M.P. Marín, L. Megías, M. Sancho-Tello, E. Fornas, J. Renau-Piqueras. Glycosylation is altered by ethanol in rat hippocampal cultured neurons. *Alcohol Alcohol.* **2006**, 41, 494-504.

53. M.E. Charness. Alcohol and the brain. *Alcohol Health Res. World.* **1990**, 14, 85–93.

54. X. Zhou, Z. Su, A. Anishkin, W.J. Haynes, E.M. Friske, S.H. Loukin, C. Kung, Y. Saimi. Yeast screens show aromatic residues at the end of the sixth helix anchor transient receptor potential channel gate. *Proc. Natl. Acad. Sci. USA*. **2007**, 104, 15555-15559.

55. F. Li, J.Z. Tsien. Memory and the NMDA receptors. *N. Engl. J. Med.* **2009**, 361, 302-303.

56. H. *Furukawa, S.K. Singh, R. Mancusso1, E. Gouaux. Subunit arrangement and function in NMDA receptors. Nature.* **2005**, *438, 185–192.*

57. *C.* Allgaier. Ethanol sensitivity of NMDA receptors. *Neurochem. Int.* **2002**, 41, 377–382.

58. K.A. Trujillo, H. Akil. Excitatory amino acids and drugs of abuse: a role for N-methyl-D-aspartate receptors in drug tolerance, sensitization and physical dependence. *Drug Alcohol Depend.* **1995**, 38, 139-154.

59. J.H. Krystal, I.L. Petrakis, G. Mason, L. Trevisan, D.C. D'Souza, N-Methyl-D-aspartate glutamate receptors and alcoholism: reward, dependence, treatment, and vulnerability. *Pharmacol Ther*. **2003**, 99, 79-94.

60. S.F. Traynelis, L.P. Wollmuth, C.J. McBain, F.S. Menniti, K.M. Vance, K.K. Ogden, R. Dingledine. Glutamate receptor ion channels: Structure, regulation and function. *Pharmacol. Rev.* **2010**, 62, 405-496.

61. P.L. Hoffman, B. Tabakoff. The role of the NMDA receptor in ethanol withdrawal. *Exp. Suppl.* **1994**, 71, 61-70.

62. K. Wirkner, W. Poelchen, L. Koles, K. Muhlberg, P. Scheibler, C. Allgaier, P. Illes. Ethanol-induced inhibition of NMDA receptor channels. *Neurochem. Int.* **1999**, 35, 153-162.

63. J.J. Woodward, R.A. Gonzales. Ethanol Inhibition of *N*-Methyl-D-Aspartate-Stimulated Endogenous Dopamine Release from Rat Striatal Slices: Reversal by Glycine. *J. Neurochem.* **1990**, 54, 712–715.

64. *B.* Givens, K. McMahon, K. Ethanol suppresses the induction of long-term potentiation in vivo. *Brain Res.* **1995**, 688, 27-33.

65. B. Givens. Low doses of ethanol impair spatial working memory and reduce hippocampal theta activity. *Alcohol. Clin. Exp. Res.* **1995**, 19, 763-767.

66. J. R. Hughes. Alcohol withdrawal seizures. *Epilepsy Behav.* **2009** 15(2), 92-97.

67. D. Ron. Signaling cascades regulating NMDA receptor sensitivity to ethanol. *Neuroscientist.* **2004**, 10, 325-336.

68. D. Ron, R.O. Messing. Signaling pathways mediating alcohol effects. *Curr. Topics Behav. Neurosci.* **2013**, 13, 87-126.

69. M. Xu, C.T. Smothers, J.J. Woodward. Effects of ethanol on phosphorylation site mutants of recombinant N-methyl-D-aspartate receptors. *Alcohol.* **2011**, 45, 373-380.

70. X. Yang, H.E. Criswell, P. Simson, S. Moy, G.R. Breese. Evidence for a selective effect of ethanol on N-methyl-D-aspartate responses: ethanol affects a subtype of the ifenprodil-sensitive N-methyl-D-aspartate receptors. *J. Pharmacol. Exp. Ther.* **1996**, 278, 114-124.

71. J. Nagy, S. Kolok, P. Dezso, A. Boros, Z. Szombathelyi. Differential alterations in the expression of NMDA receptor subunits following chronic ethanol treatment in primary cultures of rat cortical and hippocampal neurones. *Neurochem. Int.* **2003**, 42, 35-43.

72. I.A. Lobo, R.A. Harris. $GABA_A$ receptors and alcohol. *Pharmacol. Biochem. Behav.* **2008**, 90, 90–94.

73. R. Baur, F. Minier, E. Sigel. A GABA(A) receptor of defined subunit composition and positioning: concatenation of five subunits. *FEBS Lett.* **2006**, 580, 1616-1620.

74. C. R. Ravindran, M. K. Ticku. Tyrosine kinase phosphorylation of GABA(A) receptor alpha1, beta2 and gamma2 subunits following chronic intermittent ethanol (CIE) exposure of cultured cortical neurons of mice. *Neurochemical Research.* **2006**, 31, 1111-1118.

75. A.C. Grobin, S.T. Papadeas, A.L. Morrow. Regional variations in the effects of chronic ethanol administration on GABA(A) receptor expression: potential mechanisms. *Neurochemistry International*. **2000**, 37, 453-461.

76. J. M. Silvers, S. Tokunaga, G. Mittleman, D. B. Matthews. Chronic intermittent injections of high-dose ethanol during adolescence produce metabolic, hypnotic, and cognitive tolerance in rats. *Alcoholism: Clinical and Experimental Research*. **2003**, 27, 1606-1612.

77. L.G. Aguayo, R.W. Peoples, H. H. Yeh, G. E. Yevenes. GABA(A) receptors as molecular sites of ethanol action. Direct or indirect actions? *Curr. Topics Med. Chem.* **2002**, 2, 869-885.

78. A.C. Grobin, D.B. Matthews, L.L. Devaud, A.L. Morrow. The role of GABA(A) receptors in the acute and chronic effects of ethanol. *Psychopharmacol*. **1998**, 139, 2-19.

79. M. Soyka, U.W. Preuss, V. Hesselbrock, P. Zill, G. Koller, B. Bondy. GABA A2 receptor subunit gene (GABRA2) polymorphisms and risk for alcohol dependence. *J. Psychiatric Res.* **2008**, 42, 184-191.

80. S. Kumar, P. Porcu, D.F. Werner, D.B. Matthews, J. L. Diaz-Granados, R.S. Helfand, A.L. Morrow. The role of GABA(A) receptors in the acute and chronic effects of ethanol: a decade of progress. *Psychopharmacol*. **2009**, 205, 529-564.

81. C. L. Padgett, P. A. Slesinge. $GABA_B$ receptor coupling to G-proteins and ion channels, *Adv Pharmacol*. **2010**, 58, 123-147.

82. R. Lujan, F. Ciruela. $GABA_B$ receptors-associated proteins: potential drug targets in neurological disorders? *Curr. Drug Targets*. **2012**,13, 129-144.

83. N.G. Bowery, B. Bettler, W. Froestl, J.P. Gallagher, F. Marshall, M. Raiteri, S. J. Enna. International Union of Pharmacology. XXXIII. Mammalian gamma- aminobutyric acid(B) receptors: structure and function. *Pharmacol. Rev.* **2002**, 54, 247-264.

84. M. Federici, R. Nistico, M. Giustizieri, G. Bernardi, N. B. Mercuri. Ethanol enhances GABAB-mediated inhibitory postsynaptic transmission on rat midbrain dopaminergic neurons by facilitating GIRK currents. *Eur. J. Neurosci*. **2009**, 29, 1369-1377.

85. D. M. Lovinger, G. White, F. F. Wright. Ethanol inhibits NMDA-activated ion current in hippocampal neurones. *Science*. **1989**, 243, 1721-1724.

86. F. Weiss, L. J. Porrino. Behavioral neurobiology of alcohol addiction: recent advances and challenges. *The Journal of Neuroscience*. **2002**, 22, 3332-3337.

87. T. Yamaguchi, H.-L. Wang, X. Li, T. H. Ng, M. Morales. Mesocorticolimbic Glutamatergic Pathway *The Journal of Neuroscience*. **2011**, 31, 8476-8490.

88. I. Boileau, J. M. Assaad, R. O. Pihl, C. Benkelfat, M. Leyton, M. Diksic, A. Dagher. Alcohol promotes dopamine release in the human nucleus accumbens. *Synapse*. **2003**, 49, 226-231.

89. G. Di Chiara, A. Imperato. Drugs abused by humans preferentially increase synaptic dopamine concentrations in the mesolimbic system of freely moving rats. *Proceedings of the National Academy of Sciences*. **1988**, 85, 5274-5278.

90. B. Soderpalm, E. Lof, M. Ericson. Mechanistic studies of ethanol's interaction with the mesolimbic dopamine reward system. *Pharmacopsychiatry*, **2009**, 42 (Suppl 1), S87-S94.

91. M. S. Brodie, S. A. Shefner, T. V. Dunwiddie. Ethanol increases the firing rate of dopamine neurons of the rat ventral tegmental area in vitro. *Brain Research*. **1990**, 508, 65-69.

92. N. Dahmen, M. Volp, P. Singer, C. Hiemke, A. Szegedi. Tyrosine hydroxylase Val-81-Met polymorphism associated with early-onset alcoholism. *Psychiatric Genetics*. **2005**, 15, 13-16.

93. T. Sander, H. Harms, J. Podschus, U. Finckh, B. Nickel, A. Rolfs, L. G. Schmidt. Allelic association of a dopamine transporter gene polymorphism in alcohol dependence with withdrawal seizures or delirium. *Biological Psychiatry*. **1997**, 41, 299-304.

94. D. J. Hayes, A.J. Greenshaw. 5-HT receptors and reward-related behaviour: A review. *Neurosci. Biobehav. Rev.* **2011**, 35, 1419-1449.

95. D. M. Lovinger. 5-HT3 receptors and the neural actions of alcohols: an increasingly exciting topic. *Neurochem. Int.* **1999**, 35, 125-130.

96. Q. S. Yan. Extracellular dopamine and serotonin after ethanol monitored with 5 minute microdialysis. *Alcohol*. **1999**, 19, 1-7.

97. R. Feinn, M. Nellissery, H. R. Kranzler. Meta-analysis of the association of a functional serotonin transporter promoter polymorphism with alcohol dependence. *Amer. J. Med. Gen. Part B: Neuropsychiatric Genetics*. **2005**, 133, 79-84.

98. T.V.P. Bliss, G.L. Collingridge. A synaptic model of memory: Long-term potentiation in the hippocampus. *Nature*. **1993**, 361, 31–39.

99. D.M. Lovinger, G. White, F.F. Weight. NMDA receptor-mediated synaptic excitation selectively inhibited by ethanol in hippocampal slice from adult rat. *J. Neurosci.* **1990**, 10, 1372–1379.

100. J.L. Weiner, L. Zhang, P.L. Carlen. Potentiation of GABAA-mediated synaptic current by ethanol in hippocampal CA1 neurons: Possible role of protein kinase C. *J. Pharmacol. Exp. Therapeut.* **1994**, 268, 1388–1395.

101. J.L. Weiner, C.F. Valenzuela, P.L. Watson, C.J. Frazier, T.V. Dunwiddie. Elevation of basal PKC activity increases ethanol sensitivity of GABAA receptors in rat hippocampal CA1 neurons. *J. Neurochem.* **1997**, 68, 1949–1959.

102. C.F. Valenzuela, R.A. Harris. Alcohol: Neurobiology. In: J.H. Lowinson, P. Ruiz, R.B. Millman, J.G. Langrod, eds. Substance Abuse: A Comprehensive Textbook. Baltimore: Williams & Wilkins, **1997**. pp. 119–142.

103. L. Cipolotti, C.M. Bird. Amnesia and the hippocampus. *Curr. Opin. Neurol.* **2006**, 19, 593–598.

104. K.S. LaBar, R. Cabeza. Cognitive neuroscience of emotional memory. *Nature Reviews: Neuroscience*. **2006**, 7, 54–64.

105. Australian guidelines to reduce health risks from drinking alcohol: Commonwealth of Australia. National Health and Medical Research Council. **2009**.

106. M. Oscar-Berman, K. Marinkovic, Alcohol: Effects on neurobehavioral functions and the brain. *Neuropsychol. Rev.* **2007**, 17, 239-257.

107. D. Murdoch, R.O. Phil, D. Ross. Alcohol and crimes of violence: present issues. *Int. J. Addict.* **1990**, 25, 1065–1081.

108. Geetanjali, Poonam, B. Veer and R. Singh. Alcohol abuse and related health issues. *Int. Res. J. Med. Sci.*, **2016**, 4, 1-6.

Editors' Note

The effects of alcoholism on the brain, is a study of the adverse effects of ethanol or "ethyl alcohol" on brain functioning and development. The sedative and depressant effects of ethanol results in the damaging of CNS and also may lead to disfunctioning of other vital organs. Alcohol influences neurotransmitter system in the brain, memory of the addicted person, behavior etc. Although the amount of damage depend on a variety of factors like age, gender, quantity of consumption and drinking pattern, the alcoholism is a serious health risk not only for the brain but also for whole nervous system and degrades psychological condition of the individual.

❑❑❑

4

Nutritional Deficiencies and Diseases Associated with Alcoholism

Lakshna Mahajan* and Ram Singh**

Abstract

Ethanol consumption is popularly known as alcohol consumption. The alcohol consumption practice is nearly as old as human civilization. Ethanol is a known sedative and depressant. This acts on a wide range of targets such as neurotransmitter receptors and ion channels in the central nervous system. The average volume of alcohol consumed, consumption patterns, and quality of the alcoholic beverages have an impact on the mortality and morbidity related to chronic diseases and conditions. Alcoholism is also responsible for various nutritional deficiencies and diseases in humans. This chapter discusses the nutritional deficiencies and diseases associated with alcoholism.

Keywords: Alcoholism, Nutritional deficiencies, ALD, Sexual dysfunction, Infertility

INTRODUCTION

Alcohol consumption is as old as human civilization. Many chronic diseases and nutritional deficiencies are associated with alcohol

* Department of Microbiology, Swami Shraddhanand College, University of Delhi, New Delhi-110 036, India.

** Department of Applied Chemistry, Delhi Technological University, Delhi - 110 042, India.

consumption patterns such as an average volume of alcohol consumed, quality of the alcoholic beverages consumed, as well as age and sex of the consumer.[1] The health and social problems are associated with ethanol consumption in both rural and urban societies.[2-4] The problem associated is directly proportional to alcohol consumption. This prompted the World Health Organization (WHO) to pass multiple resolutions to address this issue, including the World Health Assembly's Global Strategy to reduce the harmful use of alcohol, in May 2010. The non-communicable chronic diseases and conditions are the leading diseases associated with the alcohol-attributable burden of disease.[5] In 2004, about 35 million deaths and 603 million disability-adjusted life-years (DALYs) lost were caused by chronic diseases and conditions globally.[6] Alcohol consumption was accountable for 3.4 % of the deaths and 2.4 % of DALYs.[7]

NUTRITIONAL DEFICIENCIES DUE TO ALCOHOLISM

People who are addicted to alcohol become severely deficient in necessary vitamins and minerals. The deficiency in vitamins and minerals directly affects the health of alcoholic people and expose them to many diseases. Vitamins are organic molecules with diverse roles in biochemical functions, and are essential for the normal growth and development of a multi-cellular organism. They are grouped into two categories:

(*i*) Fat soluble vitamins: Vitamins A, D, E and K.

(*ii*) Water soluble vitamins: Vitamin B complex and C

Chronic heavy alcohol drinking leads to decreased food ingestion and, impaired absorption, metabolism, and utilization; and hence is associated with deficiencies in many vitamins.[8] For example, the drinking of alcohol inhibits fat absorption and hence weaken the absorption of the fat soluble vitamins like A, D, E, and K that are usually absorbed along with dietary fats. The deficiency of vitamin A leads to night blindness whereas vitamin D deficiency is associated with softening of the bones. The deficiency of vitamin K causes delayed clotting and result in excess bleeding. Individuals who consume more than 30 percent of their calories as alcohol have the greatest risk, particularly for deficiencies in vitamin A and thiamine.

Vitamin A: Vitamin A is required for the proper functioning and development of our immune system, eyes, skin, and many other parts of our body. This is present in many foods and vegetables like liver, orange, ripe yellow fruits, leafy vegetables, carrots, pumpkin, spinach, fish, soya milk, milk, etc. According to World Health Organization (WHO), vitamin A deficiency (VAD) is the leading cause of preventable blindness in children and increases the risk of disease and death from severe infections. In pregnant women, VAD causes night blindness and may increase the risk of maternal mortality.[9]

This has been established that the chronic alcohol consumers showed deficiency in vitamin A and hence exposed to the vitamin A deficiency diseases.[10,11] The diseases like the loss of night vision (nyctalopia), xerophthalmia and blindness are associated with alcoholism.[12,13] The alcohol also has effect on hepatic vitamin A status.[14] Alcoholics showed decrease in plasma retinol levels and plasma retinol binding protein (RBP) concentrations.[15]

Thiamine: Thiamine is also known as vitamin B1 and is commonly used in combination with other Vitamin B as Vitamin B complexes.[16] This is an essential nutrient and its deficiency has fatal consequences. It has been observed that the people who are addicted to ethanol suffer from thiamine deficiency. There are several mechanisms associated with alcohol consumption that may contribute to thiamine deficiency.[16] Three important pathways involved in thiamine deficiency includes inadequate nutritional intake, reduction in absorption of thiamine from the gastrointestinal tract and reduced uptake into cells and impaired utilization of thiamine in the cells.[17]

(*a*) **Inadequate Nutritional Intake:** A healthy person requires an average of about 0.33 mg of minimum thiamine intake for every 1,000 kcal of energy that he/she consumes. The alcoholics, however, show a decreased tendency to consume thiamine at a quantity less than 0.29 mg/1,000 kcal.[18] In a study with 3,000 patients related to alcoholism, 40% showed periodic deficiency during drinking binges, while 25% exhibited prolonged thiamine deficiency, and 35% of patients showed continuous thiamine deficiency.[19] Further, it was found that there were decreased levels of thiamine monophosphate in alcoholic patients, which is a primary enzymatic conversion of thiamine required for its assimilation. On the other hand, the levels of free thiamine were found to be similar in alcoholics and control subjects.[20] This suggests the inability of the ethanol affected the person in the initial conversion of thiamine into its active, phosphate–containing form.

(*b*) **Reduction in uptake of thiamine from the gastrointestinal tract:** The studies on animals showed that in acute alcohol exposures and alcohol related deficiency diseases, alcohol interferes with the active transport of thiamine from the gastrointestinal tract. Active transport is an energy-dependent transport system that transport thiamine at low concentrations from the intestinal lumen into the blood stream and thus delivered to the cells in the body. It is carried out by a specific thiamine transporter molecule, associated with enzyme thiamine diphosphokinase (TPK) that results in the rapid addition of two phosphate groups to the thiamine once thiamine reaches inside the cell. The acute alcohol exposure interferes with the absorption of thiamine from the gastrointestinal tract at low thiamine concentrations.[21] It has been further found that the acute exposure to alcohol decreased the activity of the TPK in various tissues in a rat model up to 70% while the chronic exposure resulted in decrease up to 50% in the enzyme activity.[22] In an independent study, the ratio of phosphorylated thiamine to thiamine was significantly reduced in alcoholics than in control, suggesting that less thiamine is being phosphorylated in the alcoholics. This indirectly suggests that TPK is less active in alcoholics.[23,24]

(*c*) **Impaired thiamine utilization:** The chronic alcohol consumption affects the utilization of thiamine in the cell. This limits the availability of various cofactors associated with the activity of thiamine utilizing enzymes.[25] For example, magnesium is one of the cofactors required by thiamine–using enzymes. Magnesium is also deficient in the people with chronic alcohol consumption. Hence, deficiency of magnesium results in the thiamine deficiency. Although thiamine is available but cannot be utilized in the body, exacerbating any concurrently existing thiamine deficiency.[17]

The studies have also shown that the thiamine deficiency occurs in chronic alcoholics at a frequency ranging from a minimum of 25–31%[26,27] to 80%[28,29]. Because thiamine and the thiamine–using enzymes are present in all cells of the body, it would be plausible that inadequate thiamine affects all organ systems; however, the cells of the nervous system and heart, i.e cardiovascular system seem particularly sensitive to the effects of thiamine deficiency.

The major diseases associated with thiamine deficiency are Korasakoff's syndrome, optic neuropathy, and beriberi. A common complication associated with thiamine deficiency in chronic alcoholics is Wernicke-Korsakoff syndrome (WKS). WKS is a neuropsychiatric disorder characterized by ophthalmoplegia, ataxia and mental changes.[30] Wernicke's encephalopathy is the first part of WKS and it causes confusion, paralysis of eye nerves and difficulty with movement. Up to 90 percent of those with Wernicke's encephalopathy develop long–lasting and debilitating condition Korsakoff's psychosis, which causes memory deficits and abnormal behaviour.[31]

The other complications associated with thiamine deficiency-induced cell damage includes oxidative stress, glutamate-mediated excitotoxicity and inflammatory responses. The thiamine deficiency leads to increased production of reactive oxygen species (ROS) in the brain[32,33] as well as microglial activation[34], resulting in pathogenesis. In addition, thiamine is an essential coenzyme in various enzymatic reactions of carbohydrate metabolism, where it helps in transfer of carbon moieties in enzyme-catalyzed reactions. For example in Kreb's cycle (an important cycle for deriving energy from carbohydrates, fats and proteins) alpha-ketoglutarate dehydrogenase (α–KGDH) is a rate limiting enzyme that requires thiamine pyrophosphate for its activity. Hence, thiamine deficiency results in inefficient metabolism of carbohydrate. The inefficiency leads to oxidative stress that induces cell damage and cell death.[35,36] The lowered activity of the KGDH results in decreased energy status in the affected areas of the brain contributing to loss of neuronal function, including glutamatergic neurotransmission. This also results is increased levels of alpha-ketoglutarate leading to production of its metabolite glutamate[37] causing glutamate-mediated excitotoxicity and excitotoxic-like lesions in damaged areas of the brain. The decreased production of required metabolites from TCA cycle causes mitochondrial uncoupling, followed by mitochondrial damage ending in cell death.[38] A role of genetic predisposition to thiamine deficiency has been proposed owing to the fact that although thiamine deficiency occurs in 80 percent of alcoholics,[39] only a subset of these alcoholics develop brain disorders such as WKS. If WKS is diagnosed before severe deterioration, improving the nutrition (thiamine administration) and abstinence from alcohol has been shown to reverse impairments associated.[38]

Minerals

The chronic alcohol consumption leads to deficiencies of minerals like calcium (Ca), magnesium (Mg), iron (Fe), zinc (Zn), etc. These deficiencies are not related to alcoholism directly rather deficiencies are due to alcohol-related problems.[40,41] For example, alcoholism results in fat malabsorption leading to calcium deficiency. The magnesium deficiency occurs due to decreased intake, increased urinary excretion, vomiting, and diarrhea.[42] The gastrointestinal bleeding results in iron deficiency.[40] The mineral deficiencies can cause a variety of medical consequences from calcium-related bone disease to zinc-related night blindness and skin lesions.[43,44]

DISEASES DUE TO ALCOHOLISM

Alcoholic Liver Disease (ALD): Alcohol is associated with various liver diseases that are collectively called alcoholic liver diseases (ALD). The association between the alcohol consumption and risk of ALD has long been established. The ALD covers sets of injury that range from simple steatosis to frank cirrhosis.[45] The three histological stages of ALD includes simple steatosis (fatty liver), alcoholic hepatitis, and chronic hepatitis with hepatic fibrosis or cirrhosis.[45,46] *Cirrhosis* is a condition in which the liver is damaged and does not function properly whereas *hepatitis* is an inflammation of the liver. This has been observed that the individuals who consume alcohol more than 60 g/day develop steatosis.[47] The chronic consumption of alcohol of about 40g/day increased the risk of progression to cirrhosis to 30%, and fibrosis or cirrhosis to 37%.[48]

The effect of alcohol on the liver is also dependent on gender and age of alcoholics. For example, the women are twice more sensitive to alcohol-mediated hepatotoxicity than their male counterpart. They even develop more severe ALD at lower doses and shorter duration of alcohol consumption.[49] This may be due to the presence of differing blood alcohol levels in women in comparison to men after equal amounts of alcohol consumption.[50] The most accepted mechanism for liver damage involves the oxidative and non-oxidative breakdown of ethanol in the liver leading to the formation of free radicals, acetaldehyde, and fatty acid ethyl esters. These chemical species are responsible for damaging liver cells.[51]

Pancreatic Problem in Alcoholics: Heavy drinking can result in inflammation of the pancreas (pancreatitis). The pancreas is an organ present behind the stomach that produces digestive enzymes. The alcoholism increases the risk of acute and chronic pancreatitis.[52] The risk of developing the disease increases with both amount and duration of alcohol consumption. The combination of alcohol drinking with smoking aggravates the pancreatic problem further. The damage pathway for liver and pancreas remains almost same for the heavy chronic alcoholics.[53]

Sexual dysfunction: Chronic and persistent alcohol use is known to induce sexual dysfunction in an alcoholic person, which result in distress and interpersonal problems.[54] The sexual dysfunction (SD) is associated with many types of problems that include decreased sexual desire, difficulty in erection and achieving orgasm, sexual aversion disorder, and premature ejaculation.[55] There is a wrong believe that the consumption of alcohol before sexual intercourse improves the sexual pleasure. As per a study of 2005 by World Health Organization (WHO) across eight countries, it was found that 12% male population consumed alcohol before their first sexual intercourse.[56] However, in long and persistent alcohol abuse; some type of sexual dysfunction arises. The SD like testicular atrophy, inhibition of testosterone production, and inhibition of spermatogenesis, has been observed in the people with chronic alcohol drinking habit.[57,58] Acetaldehyde is the metabolic product of alcohol and is responsible for changing the process of testosterone production by inhibiting the enzyme protein kinase C that is involved in testosterone synthesis.[59]

Infertility: According to WHO-ICMART, infertility is a disease of the reproductive system defined by the failure to achieve a clinical pregnancy after 12 months or more of regular unprotected sexual intercourse. As per a report, one out of four couples is said to be affected by infertility. While the definitive relationship between alcohol and infertility remains to be determined, but the association of alcoholism and male/female infertility cannot be ruled out completely.[60] This has been observed that the chronic alcoholic female experienced irregularities in their menstrual cycles and ovulation and also unusual variation in the levels of estrogen and progesterone.[61-64] Infertility due to ovulatory disorders like an ovulation and oligo ovulation or endometriosis have been associated with alcohol abuse.[65] Alcoholism was found to be associated with decreased fecundability also.[66]

In the case of a male, the semen quality is associated with alcoholism.[67] The vitality, survival rate and count of sperm have dose and time effect relationship with alcoholism.[67] The alcoholic nature increases the teratozoospermia and oligozoospermia significantly.[68] The *teratozoospermia* is a condition where sperm with abnormal morphology is present whereas *oligozoospermia* refers to semen with a low concentration of sperm.

Neurological complications: The chronic and excessive alcohol consumption affect the nervous system, causing numbness and pain in hands and feet, disordered thinking, dementia, and short-term memory loss. Alcohol consumption is also associated with epilepsy, whereas alcohol withdrawal can cause seizures but not epilepsy.[69] The studies have found that a consistent dose-response relationship exists between alcohol consumption and the risk of epilepsy.[70] The heavy alcohol consumption may increase the risk of epilepsy by causing shrinkage of brain tissue (*i.e.*, cerebral atrophy).[71] The other problems associated with alcoholism include cerebrovascular infarctions, lesions, head traumas, and changes in neurotransmitter systems and ionic balances.[71,72] Another neuropsychiatric disorder linked to alcohol consumption is a unipolar depressive disorder. This disorder is found to increase two- to three-fold in alcohol-dependent people.[73]

Numerous studies also have examined the association between alcohol and Alzheimer's disease (AD) and vascular dementia.[74,75] The high alcohol consumption is considered a risk for late-onset AD.[76] A study showed a decrease in muscarinic and benzodiazepine receptors in alcoholic AD patients.[74] This has also been observed that only heavy drinkers showed neuronal cell loss whereas mild and moderate drinkers have no implication on the incidence of AD.[77] This suggested that the effect of ethanol on AD pathology only depend on the level of alcohol intake and the type of beverage consumed. The initial studied with primary neuron culture had provided information about the ability of ethanol to exacerbate Ab toxicity and neuron cell death mechanisms.[78,79]

Hematological complications: *Hematology* is the study of blood. Alcoholics are at risk for hematological complications.[80] The chronic alcohol consumption reduces the numbers of blood cells either by the suppression of hematopoiesis or due to nutritional deficiency of folic acid and other vitamins required for development of blood cells.[80] This has been established through clinical observations that the production and function of virtually all types of blood cells are adversely affected by alcohol.[81] The bone marrow of drinkers are directly affected by alcohol and leads to suppression of blood cell production. The chronic alcoholism reduces the number of blood cell precursors and causes abnormalities in these cells leading to the formation of fewer-than-normal or nonfunctional mature blood cells. This causes moderate anemia, characterized by enlarged, structurally abnormal RBC's. This also reduces numbers of WBC's, mainly neutrophils; and moderately to severely reduced numbers of platelets.[80-82]

SUMMARY

Today, society is facing the enormous burden of chronic diseases and conditions attributable to alcohol consumption. Mostly people have the misconception about the effect of drinking alcohol on their health. Alcohol has more negative impact than positive on the overall health of any individual. Starting from the brain, this affects almost all the vital organs either directly or indirectly. Alcoholic people become deficient in various essential vitamins and minerals. They develop a number of diseases associated with these deficiencies. Alcohol is also associated with various liver diseases that are collectively called alcoholic liver diseases (ALD). Alcoholic people also exposed themselves with diseases related to pancreas, sexual dysfunction, infertility and neurological complications. There is a need to get educated about the alcoholism.

ACKNOWLEDGMENTS

The author RS is thankful to Council of Scientific & Industrial Research (*CSIR*), India, for financial support.

REFERENCES

1. T. Cargiulo. Understanding the health impact of alcohol dependence. *Am. J. Health Syst. Pharm.* **2007**, 64 (5 Suppl 3), S5–11.
2. P. McGovern. *Uncorking the Past: The Quest for Wine, Beer, and Other Alcoholic Beverages.* Berkley; Los Angeles; London: The Regents of the University of California, **2009**.
3. I. Tramacere, C. Pelucchi, M. Bonifazi, *et.al.* A meta-analysis on alcohol drinking and the risk of Hodgkin lymphoma. *Eur. J. Cancer Prevent.* **2012**, 21(3), 268–273.
4. I. Tramacere, C. Pelucchi, M. Bonifazi, V. Bagnardi, M. Rota, R. Bellocco, L. Scotti, F. Islami, G. Corrao, P. Boffetta, C. La Vecchia, E. Negri. Alcohol drinking and non-Hodgkin lymphoma risk: A systematic review and a meta-analysis. *Ann. Oncol.* **2012**, *23(11), 2791-2798.*
5. J. Rehm, C. Mathers, S. Popova, M. Thavorncharoensap, Y. Teerawattananon, J. Patra. Global burden of disease and injury and economic cost attributable to alcohol use and alcohol use disorders. *Lancet.* **2009**, 373(9682), 2223– 2233.
6. World Health Organization. *GBD 2004 Summary Tables.* Geneva, Switzerland: World Health Organization; **2008**.

7. C. Parry, J. Patra, J. Rehm. Alcohol consumption and non-communicable diseases: Epidemiology and policy implications. *Addiction* **2011,** 106(10), 1718–1724.
8. WHO. Micronutrient deficiencies, **2016** (http://www.who.int/nutrition/topics/vad/en/)
9. A.M. Hoyumpa. Mechanisms of vitamin deficiencies in alcoholism. *Alcohol Clin. Exp. Res.* **1986**, 10(6), 573-581.
10. R.D. Clugston, W.S. Blaner. The Adverse Effects of Alcohol on Vitamin A Metabolism. *Nutrients.* **2012**, 4, 356-371.
11. C.S. Lieber. Relationships between nutrition, alcohol use, and liver disease. *Alcohol. Res. Health.* **2003**, 27, 220–231.
12. D.P. Roncone. Xerophthalmia secondary to alcohol-induced malnutrition. *Optometry* **2006**, 77, 124–133.
13. S.K. Majumdar, G.K. Shaw, A.D. Thomson. Vitamin A utilization status in chronic alcoholic patients. *Int. J. Vitam. Nutr. Res.* **1983**, 53, 273–279.
14. M.A Leo, C.S. Lieber. Hepatic vitamin A depletion in alcoholic liver injury. *New Engl. J. Med.* **1982**, 307, 597–601.
15. C.J. McClain, D.H. van Thiel, S. Parker, L.K. Badzin, H. Gilbert. Alterations in zinc, vitamin A, and retinol-binding protein in chronic alcoholics: A possible mechanism for night blindness and hypogonadism. *Alcohol. Clin. Exp. Res.* **1979**, 3, 135–141.
16. *L.K Mahan, S. Escott-Stump, eds. Krause's food, nutrition, & diet therapy (10th ed.). Philadelphia: W.B. Saunders Company,* **2000**.
17. G. F. Jr. Combs. The vitamins: Fundamental Aspects in Nutrition and Health (3rd ed.). Ithaca, NY: Elsevier Academic Press, **2008**.
18. J.M. Woodhill, S. Nobile. Thiamine in the 1970 Australian diet with special reference to cereals and the assessment of thiamine status. *Int. J. Vit. Nutrit. Res.* **1972**, 42, 435–443.
19. C.M. Leevy, H. Baker. Vitamins and alcoholism. *Amer. J. Clin. Nutrit.* **1968**, 21, 1325–1328.
20. C.M.E Tallaksen, T. Bohmer, H. Bell. Blood and serum thiamin and thiamin phosphate esters concentrations in patients with alcohol dependence syndrome before and after thiamin treatment. *Alcohol. Clin. Exp. Res.* **1992**, 16, 320–325.
21. A.M. Hoyumpa. Mechanisms of thiamine deficiency in chronic alcoholism. *Amer. J. Clin. Nutrit.* **1980,** 33, 2750–2761.
22. U. Laforenza, C. Patrini, G. Gastaldi, G. Rindi. Effects of acute and chronic ethanol administration on thiamine metabolizing enzymes in some brain areas and in other organs of the rat. *Alcohol Alcohol.* **1990**, 25, 591–603.

23. A.M. Hoyumpa Jr. Mechanisms of thiamin deficiency in chronic alcoholism. *Am. J. Clin. Nutr.* **1980**, 33(12), 2750-2761.

24. R.E. Poupon, G. Gervaise, P. Riant, G. Houin, J.-P. Tillement. Blood thiamine and thiamine phosphate concentrations in excessive drinkers with or without peripheral neuropathy. *Alcohol Alcohol.* **1990**, 25, 605–611.

25. G. Rindi, D. Casirola, V. Poggi, B.D. Vizia, C. Patrini, U. Laforanza. Thiamine transport by erythrocytes and ghosts in thiamine–responsive megaloblastic anemia. *J. Inher. Metab. Dis.* **1992**, 15, 231–242.

26. M. Baines. Detection and incidence of B and C vitamin deficiency in alcohol related illness. Ann. Clin. Biochem. **1978**, 15, 307-312.

27. O. Lê, M. Heroux, R.F. Butterworth. Pyrithiamine-induced thiamine deficiency results in decreased Ca(2+)-dependent release of glutamate from rat hippocampal slices. Metab. Brain Dis. **1991**, 6, 125-132.

28. J. Tang, A. Maximov, O.H. Shin, H. Dai, J. Rizo, T.C. Sudof. A complexin/ synaptotagmin 1 switch controls fast synaptic vesicle exocytosis. Cell. **2006**, 126, 1175-1187.

29. J.I. Morgan, T. Curran. Role of ion flux in the control of c-fos expression. Nature. **1986**, 322, 552-555.

30. P.W Ragan, C.K. Singleton, P.R. Martin. Brain injury associated with chronic alcoholism. CNS Spectrums. **1999**, 4(1), 66–87.

31. J.J.–L. Wang, P.R. Martin, C.K. Singleton. A transketolase assembly defect in a Wernicke–Korsakoff syndrome patient. Alcohol. Clin. Exp. Res. **1997**, 21, 576–580.

32. G.E. Gibson, H. Zhang. Interactions of oxidative stress with thiamine homeostasis promote neurodegeneration. Neurochem. Int. **2002**, 40, 493-504.

33. P. J. Langlais, G. Anderson, S.X. Guo, S.C. Bondi. Increased cerebral free radical production during thiamine deficiency. Metab. Brain Dis. **1997**, 12, 137-143.

34. K.G. Todd, R.F. Butterworth. Evidence that oxidative stress plays a role in neuronal cell death due to thiamine deficiency. J. Neurochem. **1997**, 69(Suppl), S136A.

35. K.G. Todd, R.F. Butterworth. Early microglial response in experimental thiamine deficiency: an immunohistochemical analysis. *Glia* **1999**, 25, 190-198.

36. N.Y. Calingasan, W.J. Chun, L.C. Park, K. Uchida, G.E. Gibson. Oxidative stress is associated with region-specific neuronal death during thiamine deficiency. *J. Neuropathol. Exp. Neurol.* **1999**, 58, 946-958.

37. P.J. Langlais, S.X. Zhang. Extracellular glutamate is increased in thalamus during thiamine deficiency-induced lesions and is blocked by MK-801. *J. Neurochem.* **1993**, 61, 2175-2182.

38. C.K. Singleton, P.R. Martin. Molecular mechanisms of thiamine utilization. *Curr. Mol. Med.* **2001**, 1(2), 197–207.

39. M.Y. Morgan. Alcohol and nutrition. *Brit. Med. Bull.* **1982**, 38, 21–29.

40. C.S. Lieber. Alcohol and nutrition: An overview. *Alcohol Health Res. W.* **1989**, 13(3), 197-205.

41. L. Marsano, C.J. McClain. Effects of alcohol on electrolytes and minerals. *Alcohol Health Res. W.* **1989**, 13(3), 255-260.

42. E.B. Flink. Magnesium deficiency in alcoholism. *Alcohol. Clin. Exp. Res.* **1986**, 10(6), 590-594.

43. C.J. McClain, D.R. Antonow, D.A. Cohen, S.I. Shedlofsky. Zinc metabolism in alcoholic liver disease. *Alcohol. Clin. Exp. Res.* **1986**, 10(6), 582-589.

44. L. Feinman. Absorption and utilization of nutrients in alcoholism. *Alcohol Health Res. W.* **1989**, 13(3), 207-210.

45. R.S. O'Shea, S. Dasarathy, A. J. McCullough. Practice Guideline Committee of the American Association for the Study of Liver Diseases; Practice Parameters Committee of the American College of Gastroenterology. Alcoholic Liver Disease. *Hepatology.* **2010**, 51(1), 307-328.

46. R.N. MacSween, A.D. Burt. Histologic spectrum of alcoholic liver disease. *Semin. Liver Dis.* **1986**, 6, 221-232.

47. D.W. Crabb. Pathogenesis of alcoholic liver disease: newer mechanisms of injury. *Keio. J. Med.* **1999**, 48, 184-188.

48. M.R. Teli, C.P. Day, A.D. Burt, M.K. Bennett, O.F. James. Determinants of progression to cirrhosis or fibrosis in pure alcoholic fatty liver. *Lancet.* **1995**, 346, 987-990.

49. N. Sato, K.O. Lindros, E. Baraona, K. Ikejima, E. Mezey, H.A. Jarvelainen, V.A. Ramchandani. Sex difference in alcohol-related organ injury. *Alcohol Clin. Exp. Res.* **2001**, 25, 40S-45S.

50. E. Baraona, C.S. Abittan, K. Dohmen, M. Moretti, G. Pozzato, Z.W. Chayes, C. Schaefer, C.S. Leiber. Gender differences in pharmacokinetics of alcohol. *Alcohol Clin. Exp. Res.* **2001**, 25, 502-507.

51. D.J. Tuma, C.A. Casey. Dangerous byproducts of alcohol breakdown-focus on adducts. *Alcohol Res. Health.* **2003,** 27(4), 285-290.

52. P. Chowdhury, P. Gupta. Pathophysiology of alcoholic pancreatitis: An overview. *World J. Gastroenterol.* **2006**, 12(46), 7421-7427

53. A. *Vonlaufen*, J.S. Wilson, R.C. Pirola, M.V. Apte. Role of *alcohol* metabolism in chronic pancreatitis. *Alcohol Res. Health.* **2007**, 30(1), 48-54.

54. B.S. Arackal, V. Benegal. Prevalence of sexual dysfunction in male subjects with alcohol dependence. *Ind. J. Psychiatry*. **2007**, 49(2), 109-112.

55. E.D. Moreira, D.B. Glasser, A. Nicolosi, F.G. Duarte, C. Gingell, GSSAB Investigators' Group. Sexual problems and help-seeking behaviour in adults in the United Kingdom and continental Europe. *BJU Int.* **2008**, 101, 1005-1011.

56. World Health Organization. Alcohol Use and Sexual Risk Behaviour: A Cross-Cultural Study in Eight Countries. Geneva: *World Health Organization;* **2005**.

57. R. Nordmann, C. Ribière, H. Rouach. Ethanol-induced lipid peroxidation and oxidative stress in extrahepatic tissues. *Alcohol Alcohol.* **1990**, 25, 231-237.

58. C. Rivier, S. Rivest, W. Vale. Alcohol-induced inhibition of LH secretion in intact and gonadectomized male and female rats: Possible mechanisms. *Alcohol Clin. Exp. Res.* **1992**, 16, 935-941.

59. R.A. Anderson Jr., J.M. Quigg, C. Oswald, L.J. Zaneveld. Demonstration of a functional blood-testis barrier to acetaldehyde. Evidence for lack of acetaldehyde effect on ethanol-induced depression of testosterone *in vivo*. *Biochem. Pharmacol.* **1985**, 34, 685-695.

60. S. Grover, S.K. Mattoo, S. Pendharkar, V. Kandappan. Sexual dysfunction in patients with alcohol and opioid dependence. *Ind. J. Psychol. Med.* **2014**, 36(4), 335-365.

61. P.D. Silva, J.L. Cool, K.L. Olson. Impact of lifestyle choices on female infertility. *J. Reprod. Med.* **1999**, 44, 288–296.

62. K.S. Hruska, P.A. Furth, D.B. Seifer, F.I. Sharara, J.A. Flaws. Environmental factors in infertility. *Clin. Obstet. Gynecol.* **2000**, 43, 821–829.

63. M.A. Hassan, S.R. Killick. Negative lifestyle is associated with a significant reduction in fecundity. *Fertil. Steril.* **2004**, 81, 384–392.

64. R.L. Barbieri. The initial fertility consultation: Recommendations concerning cigarette smoking, body mass index, and alcohol and caffeine consumption. *Am. J. Obstet. Gynecol.* **2001**, 185, 1168–1173.

65. F. Grodstein, M.B. Goldman, D.W. Cramer. Infertility in women and moderate alcohol use. *Am. J. Public Health.* **1994**, 84, 1429–1432.

66. T.K. Jensen, N.H.I. Hjollond, T.B. Henriksen, T. Schieke, H. Kolstad, A. Giwarcman, E. Ernst, J.P. Bonde, N.E. Skakkebaek, J. Olsen. Does moderate alcohol consumption affect fertility? Follow-up study among couples planning first pregnancy. *BMJ.* **1998**, 317, 505–510.

67. D. Gude. Alcohol and fertility. *J. Human Reprod. Sci.* **2012**, 5, 226-227.
68. D.S. Gaur, M.S. Talekar, V.P. Pathak. Alcohol intake and cigarette smoking impact of two major lifestyle factors on male fertility. *Ind. J. Pathol. Microbiol.* **2010**, 53, 35-40.
69. M. Hillbom, I. Pieninkeroinen, M. Leone. Seizures in alcohol-dependent patients: Epidemiology, pathophysiology and management. *CNS Drugs.* **2003**, 17(14), 1013–1030.
70. J.C. Ballenger, R.M. Post. Kindling as a model for alcohol withdrawal syndromes. *Brit. J. Psychiatry.* **1978**, 133, 1–14.
71. A.M. Dam, A. Fuglsang-Frederiksen, U. Svarre-Olsen, M. Dam. Late-onset epilepsy: Etiologies, types of seizure, and value of clinical investigation, EEG, and computerized tomography scan. *Epilepsia.* **1985**, 26(3), 227–231.
72. E.S. Freedland, D.B. McMicken. Alcohol-related seizures, Part-I: Pathophysiology, differential diagnosis, and evaluation. *J. Emerg. Med.* **1993**, 11(4), 463–473.
73. J. Rehm, R. Room, K. Graham, *et.al.* The relationship of average volume of alcohol consumption and patterns of drinking to burden of disease: An overview. *Addiction.* **2003**, 98(9), 1209–1228.
74. G. Freund. W.E. Ballinger. Alzheimer's disease and alcoholism: Possible interactions. *Alcohol.* 1992, 9, 233-240.
75. J. Kardos, I. Kovacs, F. Hajos, M. Kalman, M. Simonyi. Nerve endings from rat brain release copper upon depolarization. A possible role in regulating neuronal excitability. *Neurosci. Lett.* **1989**, 103, 139-144.
76. L. Fratiglioni, A. Ahlbom, M. Viitanen, B. Winblad. Risk factors for late-onset Alzheimer's disease: A population-based, case-control study. *Ann. Neurol.* **1993**, 33(3), 258-266.
77. L.E. Hebert, P.A. Scherr, L.A. Beckutt, H.H. Funkenstein, M.S. Albert, M.H. Chown, D.A. Evans. Relation of smoking and alcohol consumption to incident of Alzheimer's disease. *Am. J. Epidemiology.* **1992**, 135, 347-355.
78. A.Y. Sun, B. Draczynska-Lusiak, G.Y. Sun. Oxidized lipoproteins, beta amyloid peptides and Alzheimer's disease. *Neurotoxicity Res.* **2001**, 3, 1-12.
79. Geetanjali, Poonam, B. Veer and R. Singh. Alcohol abuse and related health issues. *Int. Res. J. Med. Sci.*, **2016**, 4, 1-6.
80. H.S. Ballard. The hematological complications of alcoholism. *Alcohol Health Res. World*, **1997**, 21, 42-52.

81. H.S. Ballard. Hematological complications of alcoholism. *Alcoholism: Clinical Exp. Res.*, **1989**, 13, 706–720.

82. J. Lindenbaum, Hematologic complications of alcohol abuse. *Seminars in Liver Dis.*, **1987**, 7, 169–181.

Editors' Note

The Chapter titled "Nutritional Deficiencies and Diseases associated with Alcoholism", explores the consequences of alcoholism that may lead to nutritional deficiencies and subsequently diseases which are a result of such deficiencies. Lack of vitamins like A, D, C, E and K lead to diseases like night blindness, softening of bones, delayed blood clotting thereby posing serious health risks for individuals addicted to alcohol. Chronic alcohol consumption also results in Alcoholic Liver Diseases (ALD) like Cirrhosis, Alcoholic Hepatitis and Steatosis and other serious health problems like Alzheimer's disease, hematological complications, pancreatic problems, sexual dysfunction and infertility. Alcohol thus, has a very serious effect on the overall health of the addicted person.

❑❑❑

5

Alcohol De-addiction: Application of Body Psychotherapies

Suhas Shetgovekar*

Abstract

Alc*oholism can be denoted as dependence on alcohol leading to addiction. Alcoholism, as is known, can have detrimental effect on one's mental and physical health. Recovery or de-addiction process is also difficult due to various factors including withdrawal symptoms. Various psychotherapies are used in order to help the affected persons deal with the situation and recover. One such group of therapies collectively known as body psychotherapies can positively contribute to the process of de-addiction. Body is an umbrella term for various psychotherapies that believe in integration of physiological or somatic, emotional, mental, spiritual and social aspects of an individual. The focus of these psychotherapies is on somatic healing and developing somatic awareness. The techniques involved in these psychotherapies mainly focus on breathing, physical movement and even touch. The present chapter thus focuses on how body psychotherapies can be applied to alcohol de-addiction. The chapter provides an introduction to body psychotherapies, covering its assumptions and principles. Various body psychotherapies have been discussed with a focus on the techniques. Further, how body*

* Discipline of Psychology, School of Social Sciences, IGNOU, New Delhi.

psychotherapies can be applied to alcohol de-addiction have also been focused on. The chapter includes discussion on the role of the psychotherapists, and the challenges and issues faced while applying body psychotherapies to alcohol de-addiction.

Keywords: Alcoholism, Alcohol De-addiction, Body Psychotherapies

INTRODUCTION

Alcoholism can be denoted as dependence on alcohol leading to addiction. It involves problems that are associated with controlling one's drinking, the person becomes preoccupied with alcohol and continues alcohol use even when it leads to problems. It also includes consumption of more alcohol so as to get the same effect and experiencing withdrawal symptoms when there is decrease or stoppage of alcohol consumption.

Alcoholism can be said to be a result of dependence that is both cognitive and physiological in nature. It can have a detrimental effect on one's mental and physical health. Regular consumption of alcohol for a considerable period of time can have severe impact on the physiology of the individual and affected person may also develop chronic disease and neurological problems. Such people are also prone to accidents that result in disability and even death. Some of the health risks involved are heart related problems, alcoholic hepatitis, cirrhosis and fibrosis of the liver, pancreatitis, cancer of the mouth, oesophagus, throat and even liver and breast. It may also lead to development of diseases like pneumonia or tuberculosis.[1]

Alcoholism can also have an impact on the overall intellectual functioning of an individual.[2] The visuospatial abilities and higher level cognitive functioning can also get affected.[3] Various higher level cognitive functioning that get affected include abstract thinking, that are mainly required in order to make plans, implement them and even change them if required.[4] Thus alcoholism can have a detrimental effect on the physiological as well as cognitive functioning of an individual. It can also affect the overall wellbeing of the individual that can then effect his/her day-to-day functioning and performance and can have a negative impact on relationship with others.

Alcoholism can be as a result of multiple causes that may include genetics, physiological factors, psychological causes and even social factors. It can also occur as a result of interaction in these factors. Thus, it can be said that whether it is causes or effects, physiological as well as psychological factors and aspects need to be focused on.

Statistical Manual of Mental Disorders, 5th edition (DSM-5)[5] under its 'Substance-Related and Addictive Disorders', Chapter 1 includes alcohol, tobacco, 'street drugs' (for example, marijuana, cocaine, inhalants besides others) and also the non-medical use/overuse of psychoactive and other prescription and nonprescription drugs (for example, ketamine, methadone, hydrocodone besides others). According to the DSM V, a "substance use disorder describes a problematic pattern of using alcohol or another substance that results in impairment in daily life or noticeable distress". The following eleven symptoms have been stated by DSM V (out of which two must be displayed within 12 months) for a persons to be diagnosed with disorder as a result of substance use[6]:

1. Consumption of alcohol or other substance more than that was planned originally.
2. Worry over stopping of the use of the substance or consistent failed efforts in this regard.
3. A large amount of time is spent in obtaining and using the drug or alcohol.
4. There is failure on the part of the person in fulfilling his/ her major duties because of use of the substance.
5. The person will experience craving for the substance, whether drug or alcohol.
6. There is continued use of substance, despite of health problems, caused or worsened due to substance consumption. The effect can be on both mental and physical health.
7. The consumption of substance is continued despite of its negative effect on the relationship of person with others.
8. The substance is repeatedly used even in dangerous situations.
9. Use of drug or alcohol leads to giving up or reduction of persons activities.
10. There is building up of tolerance to the substance. As defined by DSM V, tolerance is "either needing to use noticeably larger amounts over time to get the desired effect or noticing less of an effect over time after repeated use of the same amount."

11. Withdrawal symptoms like anxiety, fatigue, nauseam irritability and even hand tremor, seizures with regard to alcohol are experienced by the person when the use of the substance is stopped.

It is important to note these symptoms as on the basis of these suitable body psychotherapy techniques can be provided to the person with alcoholism. This application can be during the de-addiction process as well as in order to avoid a relapse.

Alcohol de-addiction is a process through which a person with alcoholism is provided help to recover. The process of alcohol de-addiction is not an easy one. This recovery or de-addiction process is difficult due to various factors including withdrawal symptoms. Further, there are possibilities of relapses as well. There are various ways of alcohol de-addiction, including, medical approaches and psychological treatments. There are other ways as well that mainly focus on the sociocultural aspects towards such a treatment. And most often a combination of such approaches is necessary to help the person deal with alcoholism.

Psychotherapy is most often used to help the person deal with behaviour problems accompanying alcoholism. Cognitive Behaviour Therapy, for example, has been effectively used to treat alcoholism.[7,8,9] In the present discussion, the main focus will be on a type of psychotherapy that is termed as Body Psychotherapy.

BODY PSYCHOTHERAPIES

Various psychotherapies, as discussed above, are used in order to help the affected persons deal with the situation and recover. One such group of therapies collectively known as body psychotherapies can positively contribute to the process of de-addiction.

Body psychotherapies is an umbrella term for various psychotherapies that believe in integration of physiological or somatic, emotional, mental, spiritual and social aspects of an individual. The main focus of these psychotherapies is on somatic healing and developing somatic awareness.

Body psychotherapy was proposed by William Reich. Though, the origin of body psychotherapy can also be traced to Sigmund Freud, when in 1923 he stressed the significance of body psychoanalysis.[10] It was further researched by Reich who felt that counselling or mere talk therapy was not sufficient in order to reinstate the energy flow, that gets blocked as a person is growing up, due to the defence that are developed in order to avoid emotions that are painful in nature. These defences were termed by Reich as 'Muscular Armouring', a kind of muscle tension. Reich also felt that the emotional blockages can be removed by applying pressure (by touch) to the muscles.[10]

The term 'Body Psychotherapy' was coined by European Association of Body Psychotherapy (EABP) in the year 1991.[11] Body psychotherapies are also referred to as somatic psychotherapies. The field of body psychotherapy is eclectic to greater extend and includes various approaches, perspectives and techniques and to greater extent are experiential in nature. Body Psychotherapy in a way originated from psychoanalysis, but also displays a humanistic perspective (as in case of Chiron Body Psychotherapy). Thus this therapy to a greater extent brings about an integration of psychodynamic and person entered approaches.[12]

The European Association for Body Psychotherapy (EABP), defines body psychotherapy as "a distinct branch of Psychotherapy, well within the main body of Psychotherapy, which involves a different and explicit theory of mind–body functioning which takes into account the complexity of the intersections and interactions between the body and the mind. The common underlying assumption is that the body is the whole person and there is a functional unity between mind and body. Many other approaches in Psychotherapy touch on this area. Body Psychotherapy considers this fundamental".[13]

Yet another definition, by European Association for Psychotherapy defines Body psychotherapy as "a distinct 'mainstream' branch of psychotherapy within the field of psychotherapy, which has a long history and a large body of literature and knowledge based upon a sound theoretical position. It involves a different and explicit theory of mind-body functioning which takes into account the complexity of the intersections and interactions between the body and the mind. The common underlying assumption is that the body is the whole person and there is a functional unity between the mind and the body. The body does not merely mean the "soma" and that this is, in some way, separate from the mind, the "psyche". Many other approaches in psychotherapy touch on this area (for example, psychosomatics). Body Psychotherapy is different in that it considers this unity as paramount and fundamental. Any approach to the mind therefore involves the body as well, de facto; and every aspect of the body, affects and is affected by the mind, and not just the brain".[14]

As is apparent from both these definitions, body psychotherapies mainly focuses on both mind and body. Further, it also highlights the interaction between body and mind. One's body can be described as a gateway or an opening to one's unconscious emotions and feelings. These unconscious emotions and feelings can then be expressed through our body in terms of bodily movements, gestures, expressions and even voice. The main assumption of body psychotherapies is that there exists a functional unity between the psychological and physiological aspects of a human being and thus a relationship exists between the psychological processes and somatic manifestations. The techniques involved in these psychotherapies mainly focus on breathing, physical movement and even touch.

There are various body psychotherapies that are available today. To name a few, Chiron Body Psychotherapy (by Lowen and Pierrakos), Hakomi (by Ron Kurtz), Bioenergetic Analysis (by Alexander Lowen), Rolfing's Structural Integration (by Ida Pauline Rolf), Postural integration (by Jack Painter), Body-Mind Centering (Bonnie Bainbridge Cohen), Body-Mind Psychotherapy (by Susan Aposhyan), Biodynamic Psychology (by Greda Boyesen), Biosynthesis (by David Boadella) and Integrative Body Psychotherapy (by Jack Rosenberg). All these therapies have a common thread in terms of their focus on body and mind and the connection between the two, besides the assumption regarding a person's relationship with his/her own self, with others and world as a whole that ingrained not only in one's thoughts and mind but also in one's body.[15] These therapies to a greater extent share certain theoretical concepts. Most of these psychotherapies emphasize on the experiences that are somatic in nature, they also discuss about development of body-ego. Embodied mind theory is also focused on by most of these psychotherapies. They further deal with regulation of emotions, bodily processes and body memory systems.[16] The body is also seen as 'a means of exploration and communication'.[17]

Though most of these body psychotherapies have their own approach, Nick Totton has stated three approaches to this psychotherapy, namely the Adjustment model, the Trauma/ Discharge model and the Process Model,[18] discussed as follows:

Adjustment Model: This mainly deals with body and thus involves techniques that focus on releasing the blocked energy in the body. Examples are the psychotherapies by Rolfing and Postural Integration that include painful deep tissue work and biodynamic massage which involves gentle massage. The techniques related to body reeducation can also be included under this.

Trauma/Discharge Model: According to this model, the focus of the techniques need to be on the reflexes that are not expressed and also completion of reflexes that have not been released. Such techniques could help in dealing with the trauma in the body as a result of neglect (chronic), traumatic experiences and abuse and so on.

Process Model: This model has been influenced by Jung, Gestalt psychology and Existential psychology. It mainly involves techniques related to movement, gestures, and even ideas and images, that help to promote awareness as well as enhance expression. The model mainly focuses on the body as well as the symptoms displayed, and the story embodied by these.

The nature, approaches and principles of body psychotherapies make them suitable for application to alcohol de-addiction process. The next section discusses the application of body psychotherapies to alcohol de-addiction.

APPLICATION OF BODY PSYCHOTHERAPIES TO ALCOHOL DE-ADDICTION

Body psychotherapies have a large scope of application from self and somatic awareness to dealing with anxiety, stress and depression. Body psychotherapies were found to be effective with regard to existential and psychological problems like physical, sexual, mental and quality of life, besides suicide prevention amongst the clients that were studied.[19] These can also be adequately applied to mental disorders like schizophrenia from psychosis, mania, anxiety and depressive disorders as well as personality disorders.[20]

Body psychotherapies can have a significant contribution to alcohol de-addiction process and relapse due to it's focus on both body and mind. The suitability of body psychotherapies in the de-addiction process lies in both psychological and physical basis of alcoholism, in terms of causal factors as well as effects. The symptoms of alcoholism also are both cognitive as well as physiological in nature. This again makes the application of body psychotherapy more relevant.

Research on the effect of body-mind treatment component on alcoholic inpatients was carried out by Ernalinski *et al* (1997).[21] In the study, a group of persons with alcoholism were provided with physical fitness program in addition to the usual treatment provided. The group of persons with alcoholism displayed less craving for alcohol when they were compared with the group that was provided just the standard treatment. Studies by Collingwood and Willett (1971)[22] also indicated that training with regard to physical fitness leads to changes in attitude towards self, one's body and leads to self acceptance.

There are various techniques in body psychotherapies. Most often these techniques involve breathing and movement besides touch. Relaxation techniques are also used in order to become more aware and mindful about one's physical aspect, to develop physical awareness and enhance expression of emotions. Breathing is also used to a greater extent to promote deeper awareness. Body psychotherapies (For example, IBP) also include a number of exercises and body movements that can have a positive impact on the persons with alcoholism. To add, most of the body psychotherapies also work on relationship that can again be significant in the case of alcoholism, where a person with alcoholism face issues and problems in their relationship (Integrative Body Psychotherapies are frequently used with couples). Thus, its principles and techniques can also be applied in case of persons with alcoholism in order to help them enhance their relationship. Focusing on relationship is also important, in a way, to garner support from others that can have a positive impact on his/her recovery and reduce the chances of relapse.

Though not much of research is available on the application of body psychotherapies to alcohol de-addiction, few studies have been discussed here. Thus, significant research needs to be carried out and promoted in this direction to recognise the role that body psychotherapies can play in the de-addiction process.

Certain techniques of body psychotherapies are discussed further for their possible application to alcohol de-addiction process. One of the body psychotherapies is Bioenergetic Analysis, that is mainly based on the continuity that exists between the body and the mind. It was proposed by Lowen. Bioenergetics analysis can be effectively used in order to deal with chronic muscle tensions and also manage emotions. Some of the techniques of Bioenergetics are body scan, explorations of your breathing pattern, grounding and connecting to the Earth, centering and being present, movements with an emotional and bioenergetic flavour, attachments and connections to other people, the emotions and the process of healing.[23] Most often the bioenergetic exercises go along with the practice of mindfulness as well. Such techniques can be used during alcohol de-addiction process to help persons develop self and somatic awareness.

Mindfulness is one of the prominent techniques under Body Psychotherapies. Self awareness and acceptance of self in a non judgemental manner is basic to mindfulness, which can help an individual towards healing. Practicing an exercise like mindfulness can be of help during de-addiction process or even in order to prevent relapse. A study in this context was carried out by Bowen *et al* (2009)[24] to evaluate the effectiveness of Mindfulness-Based Relapse Prevention (MBRP) program (as a post care approach after the completion of an intensive treatment for substance use disorder) in comparison with the treatment as usual (TAU). Randomised controlled trial was used in the study. The results indicated positive effect of MBRP when compared with TAU. There was also decreased craving and increased acceptance amongst the participants. Exercises like body scan helps develop awareness about one's body. It can help an individual not only develop mindfulness but also uncover deeper aspects of oneself. An exercise like body scan will help in acceptance of one's body. These exercises and techniques can be effectively used for persons with alcoholism in order to help them become more aware about their own body and physiological symptoms and deal with them.

Hakomi is another body psychotherapies that can be effectively used with issues including anxiety, depression and even substance abuse and addiction. It can also be used to deal with stress, physical tension (chronic) and relationship problems. These are some of the symptoms displayed by a person with alcoholism and thus techniques of Hakomi can be effectively used to help deal with such symptoms. The basis of Hakomi is that there exist a large amount of information (including physical and emotional pain, trauma and even happy and sad memories) in one's body. These are then manifested in form of various physical and psychological problems. The therapeutics processed thus include a combination of techniques like mindfulness, unity, mind body integration and so on. Mindfulness, for example, is one of the techniques that can help the person become aware of their internal experiences and help in the process of self discovery. Mindfulness can be effectively used in healing such persons. The technique of Assisted Self Discovery of Hakomi method can be used to help persons with substance abuse.[25]

Rebirthing is yet another technique used under body psychotherapies that can be effectively used for people with alcoholism. This is a technique developed by Leonard Orr in 1970s. A study was carried out by Rajski (2002),[26] focused on the assumptions and practicality of using breathing, known as Rebirthing for people who are addicted to alcohol. The results indicated that the sobriety rate as declared by self after one year program was more than 50%.

There is also Integrative Body Psychotherapy (IBP), found by Dr. J. L. Rosenberg, that can be effectively used in alcohol de-addiction. IBP involves an integration of various therapies like objection relation therapy, gestalt therapy, Reichian therapies, analytical therapies as well as eastern practices. The fundamental goal of IBP is helping an individual in reviving ones core self, which can then be sustained by dealing with mind-body disturbances. The focus of IBP is on person's participation, self responsibility, management of stress and lifestyle, affect regulation and mind-body healing. Further, it also focuses on the core sense of self and wellness. IBP techniques involve breath work, body work and also include talk therapy.[27]

The principles and techniques of body psychotherapies can be applied in alcohol de-addiction process in the following ways:

1. Since the main focus of the body psychotherapies is on both body and mind, they can be adequately applied to alcoholism that has both physiological and psychological impact. Such techniques will help person deal with worry, anxiety, irritation as well with various health related problems.
2. The techniques related to breathing, movement and touch can be adequately used to help persons with alcoholism become more self aware as well as aware about their bodies and this can help them recover faster. Mindfulness, for example, can help such persons to understand their inner experiences and lead them towards self discovery.
3. It can also help such persons deal with withdrawal symptoms. Breathing, rebirthing and various relaxation techniques can be effectively used in this regard.
4. Regular practice of techniques of body psychotherapies can also help in avoidance of relapse.

5. Techniques of body psychotherapies can help persons deal with their relationship issues.
6. Continued practice of techniques of body psychotherapies can also have health benefits and can be used to promote overall wellbeing.
7. Body psychotherapies can be administered to individual persons as well as group, based on the requirement of the situation and the treatment.
8. Family of the person with alcoholism plays an important role. Other family member can also be taught about body psychotherapies techniques so that they can practice them regularly and are able to develop self and somatic awareness. This will help them deal with their psychological issues and provide better support to the person undergoing de-addiction process.
9. The techniques of body psychotherapies can also be administered in a group. These are referred to as Body Group Psychotherapies. Though a few techniques require to be practiced individually and for which certain amount of privacy is also required as the person reflects about his/her feelings.
10. Body psychotherapies can also be used effectively in combination with other psychotherapies and even other treatment approaches, as is common in alcohol de-addiction process.

Psychotherapist plays a significant role in application of body psychotherapies, as is the case with any other psychotherapies. However, in case of body psychotherapies, the role is even more significant as the therapist needs be adequately trained and should possess the necessary skills and expertise in body psychotherapy/ies. Some of the body psychotherapies also require the therapist to play a role of an educator, where he/she has to teach the techniques to the person. Attention also needs to be payed to the non verbal communication and behavior of the person. The therapeutic relationship is also very important in order to build the trust between the therapist and the person. Which in turn is relevant to encourage and promote sincere effort and dedication on the part of the person while he/she practices the techniques or exercises. The therapist also plays an important role in creating a safe environment in which the healing process of the person can be initiated (for example, in Bioenergetics). Case history and diagnosis also needs to be carried out in order to determine a suitable plan of action and identify the specific techniques of body psychotherapies that need to be used with the person. Psychotherapist also have to supervise the person, especially, at the initial stage.

Despite of its effectiveness, there are numerous challenges that a psychotherapist can face while practicing body psychotherapies. Any psychotherapist interested in practicing body psychotherapies needs to acquire required expertise and practice. Further, the person undergoing de-addiction also needs to be serious, willing and dedicated towards practicing the techniques of body psychotherapies as this therapy requires active involvement on part of the person. Body psychotherapies can be time consuming as well as lengthy which can be a challenge. The outcome may also not be quick. Thus again it will require persistence and patience on the part of the therapist and the person.

Utmost care needs to be taken by the psychotherapist while selecting a body psychotherapy or techniques. This needs to be done only after obtaining detailed information about the person. It is possible that certain techniques may not be suitable for certain persons and the same needs to be avoided, thus the significance of adequate training in body psychotherapy/ies is stressed again.

Further, some of the body psychotherapies also involve touch in various of its techniques. Practicing such techniques can put counsellors and psychotherapists in trouble as touching can be seen as an unethical behaviour.[28] Though use of touch by a professional after extensive training is considered as ethical.[29,30] Therapists practicing such techniques need to be adequately aware of the ethical issues of the place/State/Country they are practicing in and also need to acquire necessary expertise.

CONCLUSION

Body psychotherapies thus with focus on both body and mind can be effectively used in alcohol de-addiction process. Various techniques under varied body psychotherapies can be used based on the symptoms displayed by the person with alcoholism. Though, there is a paucity of research in application of body psychotherapies in the process of alcohol de-addiction, the chapter discussed few studies that highlight the positive impact of certain techniques of body psychotherapies. Research in this direction also needs to be promoted. The psychotherapists plays an important role in application of body psychotherapies and there are various challenges as well, mainly related to the ethical issues, that need to be adequately addressed.

REFERENCES

1. Stevens. (**2013**). Understanding Addiction to Alcohol. Retrieved November 30th, 2015 from https://www.bhpalmbeach.com/sites/default/files/eBooks/understanding_addiction_to_alcohol.pdf.
2. O. A. Parsons. Neurocognitive deficits in alcoholics and social drinkers: A continuum? Alcohol *Clinical and Experiential Research*, **1998**, 22(4), 954-96.
3. M. Oscar-Berman, B. Shagrin, D. L. Evert, C. Epstein. Impairments of Brain and Behavior: The neurological Effects of Alcohol. *Alcohol Health Research World*, **1997**, 21(1), 65-75.
4. P. R. Giancola, H. B. Moss. Executive Cognitive Functioning in Alcohol Use Disorders. In *Recent Developments in Alcoholism*, **1998**, 14, 227-51.
5. Substance-related and addictive disorders. In Diagnostic and Statistical Manual of Mental Disorders. 5th ed. Arlington, Virginia.: American Psychiatric Association; **2013**. Retrieved June 13th, 2015 from http://www.psychiatryonline.org.
6. J. Medina. (**2015**). Symptoms of Substance Use Disorders (Revised for DSM-5). Psych Central. Retrieved November 30, 2015 from http://psychcentral.com/disorders/revised-alcoholsubstance-use-disorder/.
7. P. M. Monti, D. B. Abrams, R. M. Kadden, N. L. Cooney. Treating Alcohol Dependence: A C oping Skills Training Guide in the Treatment of Alcoholism. Guilford: New York, **1989**.
8. T. Beck, F. D. Wright, C. F. Newman, B. S. Liese. Cognitive Therapy of Substance Abuse. Guilford: New York, **1993**.
9. M. D. Litt, R. M. Kadden, N. L. Cooney, E. Kabela. Coping Skills and Treatment Outcomes in Cognitive–Behavioral and Interactional Group Therapy for Alcoholism. *J. Consulting Clinical Psychology*.**2003**, 71(1), 118-28.
10. H. Ellis. A Matter of Mind and Body. Retrieved November 30th, 2015 from http://somaticpsychotherapy.com.au/index.php?option=com_content&task=view&id=48&Itemid=45
11. Eiden. Application of Post- Reichan Body Psychotherapy: A Chirion Perspective. In Body Psychotherapy, Tree Staunton, Ed, Routledge: New York, **2012**.
12. M. Soth. Current Body Psychotherapy: An Integral- Relational Approach for 21st century? *Therapy Today*, **2005**, 16, 9.
13. N. Totton. Body Psychotherapy: An Introduction. Open University Press:USA, **2003**.

14. http://www.europsyche.org/contents/13215/body-psychotherapy assessed on 19th November, 2015.

15. Bloch-Atefi, J. Smith. The effectiveness of body-oriented psychotherapy: A review of the literature. PACFA: Melbourne, **2014**.

16. F. Röhricht. Body-Oriented Psychotherapy–the State of the Art in Empirical Research and Evidence Based Practice: a Clinical Perspective. *J. Body, Movement and Dance in Psychotherapy*, **2009**, 4(2), 135-156.

17. M. C. Heller. Body psychotherapy. History, concepts, methods. W.W. Norton & Co.New York.,**2012**.

18. T. Brown. (**2015**). Body Psychotherapy – a short guide to the art and science of Bodylistening. Retrieved December 2nd, 2015 from http://www.bodyworks.org.uk/body_psychotherapy.htm.

19. S. Allmer, I. Ventegodt, K. J. Merrick. Positive effects, side effects, and adverse events of clinical holistic medicine: A review of Gerda Boyesen's nonpharmaceutical mind-body medicine (biodynamic body-psychotherapy) at two centers in the United Kingdom and Germany.International *Int. J. Adolescent Medicine and Health.* **2009**, 21(3), 281-297.

20. F. Röhricht. Body psychotherapy for the Treatment of Severe Mental Disorders: An Overview, *Body, Movement and Dance in Psychotherapy: An Int. J. Theory, Res.Practice*, **2015**, 10 (1), 51-67

21. R. Ermalinski, P. G. Hanson, B. Lubin, J. I. Thornby, P. A. Nahormek. Impact of a Body- Mind Treatment Component on Alcoholic Inpatients. *J Psychosocial Nursing and Mental Health Services*, **1997**, 35(7), 39-45.

22. L. Willett and R. Collingwood,. The Effects of Physical Training upon Self-concept and Body Attitude. *J. Clinical Psychology*, **1971**, 27(3), 411–412.

23. What is Bioenergetics? Retrieved November 29th, 2015 http://www.bioenergetic-therapy.com.

24. S.W. Bowen, N. Chawla, S.E. Collins, K. Witkiewitz, S. Hsu, J. Grow, S. Clifasefi. M. Garner, A. Douglass, M. E. Larimer, A. Marlatt. Mindfulness-based relapse prevention for substance use disorders: A pilot efficacy trial. *Substance Abuse*,**2009**, 30(4), 295-305.

25. Martin. Working with Addictions.Retrieved November, 30th, 2015 from http://www.mindfulsomatictherapy.com/working-with-addiction-the-hakomi-way.html.

26. P. Rajski. Therapeutic use of breathing with people addicted to alcohol in the program "Rebirthers for Alcoholics", Siemianowice, Poland. *Int. J. Advancement of Counselling*, **2002**, 24, 123-136.

27. J. L. Rosenberg, B. K. Morse. Integrative Body Psychotherapy. http://www.ibponline.org/resources/Couples_Therapy.pdf assessed on 25th November, 2015.

28. American Counseling Association ACA (**1996**). American Counseling Association Code of Ethics and Standards of Practice. Retrieved 20th November, 2015 from http://www.cacd.org/codeofethics.html.

29. M. Hunter, J. Struve. The Ethical Use of Touch in Psychotherapy. Sage Publications.: California, **1998**.

30. United States Association of Body Psychotherapists (**2004**). Link to Body Psychotherapy National/International Associations. Retrieved November 20th, 2015 from http://www.usabp.org/.

Editors' Note

The chapter "Alcohol de-addiction: application of body psychotherapies" deals with different de-addiction techniques/processes available to combat the habit of alcoholism. The use of body-psychotherapies in de-addiction of an alcoholic person is the special focus of the chapter. Since this therapy involves combining of body and mind aspects in the healing process, it can play an important role in de-addiction process either standalone or in combination with other therapies. Body-psychotherapies like Bio-energetic Analysis, Mindfulness, Hakomi and Rebirthing have been discussed and evaluated as possible alternatives in treating addiction. However, certain issues like expertise in such techniques, ethical issues, and adequate information about the addicted person should be kept in mind while using body-psychotherapies.

❑❑❑

6

Understanding the Role of Probiotics as a Possible Treatment Strategy for Alcoholism Induced Liver Dysfunction

Sriram Seshadri*

Abstract

Alcohol consumption has been long associated with various morbidities and even mortality. Alcoholic fatty lever disease (AFLD) results from excessive alcohol consumption. Various liver disease such as NASH, NAFLD, AFLD, fibrosis and cirrhosis share common background i.e. low grade chronic inflammation. It is likely that the gut microbiota is involved in a complex metabolic modulation and the translocation of gut microflora may also contribute to maintaining the low-grade inflammatory status in various liver disease and metabolic disorder. The probiotics is safer and cheaper alternative to modulate gut microbiota. In this chapter we describe the role of gut bacteria in liver pathophysiology and use of probiotics as therapeutic target. Probiotics not only just maintain balance of bacteria but also have positive impact on gut permeability, and thus reduces endotoximia.

Keywords: Gut Microbiota, Probiotics, Liver Inflammation, Cirhosis, antibiotics, CLD

* Institute of Science, Nirma University, SG Highway, Chharodi, Ahmedabad, Gujarat, India.

INTRODUCTION

While consumed responsibly and carefully, alcohol can be loved without repercussions. Unfortunately, whilst consuming becomes a trouble the consequences can be disastrous for the fitness of the human frame. Consistent with the countrywide Institute on Alcohol Abuse and Alcoholism, the instant outcomes of alcohol including an increase in blood alcohol attention can begin 10 minutes after your first sip. However, it's the long time outcomes alcohol may have at the frame which you need to be greater concerned approximately. Research shows that excessive alcohol intake can result in a selection of various cancers consisting of mouth, esophagus, throat, liver, and breast. It could also cause severe damage to nearly all the body's predominant organs.[1]
Current studies have reported that characteristic antioxidants present in a glass of red wine decreased the risk of cardiovascular disease. But, excessive alcohol intake starts to weaken the coronary heart muscle ensuing irregularities in blood flow. Alcoholics and binge drinkers are regularly encountered by cardiomyopathy in which the coronary heart stretches and droops. Human beings diagnosed with cardiomyopathy as a result of alcohol generally tend to revel in shortness of breath, arrhythmia (irregular heartbeat), fatigue, enlarged liver, and a chronic cough. Alcohol also can aggrevate the chance of a coronary heart attack, stroke, and high blood pressure.

Alcohol could have a destructive effect on the neuropsychology and brain functioning. It slows the relay of signals among neurotransmitters. The ethanolic content in the alcoholic drinks can damage multiple areas of the brain. Long term detrimental effects of altered brain neurotransmitters includes behavioral and functional modifications which include melancholy, tension, memory loss, and seizures. Alcoholism combined with bad diet regimn can also trigger Wernicke-Korsakoff syndrome or "wet mind". Alcoholics with "wet mind" suffers from a state of despair characterised by means of reminiscence loss, confusion, hallucinations, loss of muscle coordination, and an inability to shape new recollections and memories.

In line with the effect on the brain, excess alcohol results in secretion of pancreatic enzymes internally rather than its release into the small intestines. This accumulation of enzymes within the pancreas leads to inflammation. The pancreatic inflammation or pancreatitis, can both occur as a sudden attack (acute pancreatitis) that includes symptoms such as abdominal pain, nausea or vomiting, increase heart rate, diarrhea, and fever or chronic pancreatitis which slowly deteriorates the pancreas, resulting in diabetes or even loss of life.

The diuretic effects alcohol includes increased quantity of urine produced by the body. The kidneys aren't able to do their job of regulating the flow and makeup for the body fluids along with the distribution of sodium, potassium, and chloride ions. This may in turn disturb our stability of electrolytes. Excess alcohol consumption also can lead to high blood pressure, which is the second leading reason of kidney failure.

The importance of liver has been in general underplayed. Liver tends to modulate proper digestion of food, nutrient absorption, controls infections, and detoxification of toxins from the body. There are over two million people residing in the U.S. who suffer from liver ailment due to excessive alcohol consumption. Liver cirrhosis ranked because the twelfth leading motive of demise among Americans in 2009. Out of the 31,522 deaths reported annually, 48% were alcohol related. Approximately one out every three liver transplants in the U.S. is resultant of liver damage caused by alcohol intake.

Liver play a precise and unique role in glucose metabolism through glucose breakdown, as glycogen reserviour, or synthesis in Hepatocytes. It has role in cleansing of harmful materials. It is the principal regulator for lipid metabolism having primary function in synthesis and degradation of fatty acid.[2] In accord with its crucial role in power homeostasis, disease affecting it, are also quite complicated and alters its core metabolic pathway.

The diversity of liver diseases includes alcoholic liver disorder, non alcoholic fatty liver disease (NAFLD), liver cirrhosis, cancer and hepatitis. There are three major types of alcohol-associated liver disease: alcoholic fatty liver disease, alcoholic hepatitis, and alcoholic cirrhosis.

ALCOHOLIC FATTY LIVER DISEASE

Alcoholic fatty liver disease is resultant of deposition of fats in liver cells. It acts as a precursor for the onset of alcohol-associated liver disease. There are usually no symptoms associated. If any symptoms do occur, they may include fatigue, weakness, and discomfort localized to the right top stomach. Liver enzymes levels may be increased, however tests of liver characteristics are generally normal. Most of the heavy drinkers have fatty liver disease. Alcoholic fatty liver disease may be reversible when the individual concerned abstains from alcohol consumption.

ALCOHOLIC HEPATITIS

Alcoholic hepatitis is characterised by fats deposition in liver cells, associated with inflammation and moderate scarring of the liver. Symptoms include loss of appitite, nausea, vomiting, abdominal pain, fever and jaundice. Liver enzymes are highly elevated and examination of liver function shows high level of abnormalities. Up to 35 % of heavy drinkers have high incidence of alcoholic hepatitis and of those 55 % have cirrhosis co-associated with it. Alcoholic hepatitis may be moderate or severe. Moderate alcoholic hepatitis can be reversed following abstinence while severe alcoholic hepatitis can occur all of sudden and results in critical complications consisting of liver failure and death.

ALCOHOLIC CIRRHOSIS

Alcoholic cirrhosis, the most advanced kind of alcohol mediated liver injury that is characterized by severe or intense scarring and disruption of the normal histoarchitecture of the liver. The hard scar tissue replaces soft healthy tissue. Around 10-20 % of heavy drinkers develop cirrhosis. Symptoms of cirrhosis can be like those of intense alcoholic hepatitis. Cirrhosis is the most severe form of alcohol-associated liver disorder and is not reversed upon abstinence. However, abstinence might also improve the signs and symptoms and signs of liver disorder and prevent in addition damage.

Alcohol intake increases the intestinal permeability to a variety of substances that encompass bacterial endotoxins, such as lipopolysaccharide.[3] Lipopolysaccharide 'sensitises' Kupffer cells by binding with the CD14 receptor. This binding activates the nuclear factor - kappa β (NF-kβ) which, in turn, causes increased transcription of pro-inflammatory cytokines such as TNF-α, IL-6 and transforming growth factor beta (TGF-β)[3-5]. TNF-α and IL-6 are specially involved in cholestasis and synthesis of acute-phase proteins, while TGF-β may be significantly involved in fibrogenesis thru the activation of hepatic stellate cells. The final scenario should be characterized by means of necro-inflammation, apoptosis and fibrosis, which leads to the development and progression of liver diesase, finally culminating in cirrhosis (Figure 1).

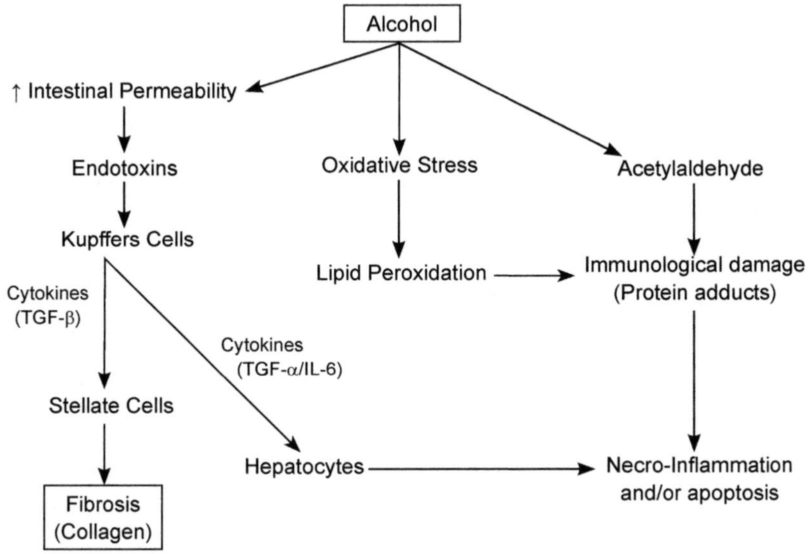

Fig. 1 Mechanism of Alcohol-induced hepatic damage

The liver is susceptible to exposure of bacterial products which gets translocated from intestine lumen thru portal vein, is accountable for liver inflammation. Bacterial product translocation is caused by altered permeability due to bacterial over hauling and alteration in intestinal microfloral composition. These translocated micro organisms and/or bacterial products *i.e.* LPS and Peptidoglycan induce liver inflammation thru activation of Toll like receptors (TLR) and NOD-like receptors (NLR)[6-7]. Obesity and type 2 diabetes (T2D) are also associated with inflammation and activation of immune system mechinary thru intestine metabolites like free fatty acids (FFA), lipids and infiltration of bacterial products like LPS, leading to development of diseases or disorders.[8]

Alcohol-induced liver disease (AILD) is one of the most common and lethal causes of chronicliver disease.[9] Various demographic and population based studies have raised a concern that both the prevalence and the severity of AILD may be rising in association with the obesity epidemic. Obesity appears to aggravate all intermediate stages of AILD, which includes alcoholic fatty liver, alcoholic steatohepatitis, and alcoholic cirrhosis.[10-12]

LIVER AND ADIPOSE TISSUE

There is an established interaction between liver and adipose tissue in regulating fat homeostasis. Adipose tissue is involved in a dual function, it is involved in the synthesis of fatty acids which is delivered to the liver and acts as a storage depot for triglycerides that are produced by liver and subsequently released into the bloodstream. It has now becone clearly evident that adipose or the fat also plays a crucial and vital role in regulating the intermediary metabolism and immunity through the production of numerous pluripotent soluble factors, which includes adipokines (*e.g.*, leptin, resistin, and adiponectin), neurotransmitters (*e.g.*, norepinephrine, neuropeptide Y, and angiotensin II), and cytokines [*e.g.*, tumor necrosis factor-alpha (TNF-α) and interleukin-6].[13-14] Thus, adipose tissue is an essential neuroendocrine organ, playing an important role in the immunological responses and activation.

In genetically modified mice, the fatty acid biosynthesis was promoted via activation of sterol regulatory element-binding protein-1 (SREBP-1). Activation of SREBP-1 is associated with hepatic fat accumulation.[15] Pathogenesis of alcoholic fatty liver is associated with elevated hepatic fatty acid biosynthesis which is relative to fatty acid oxidation. It has been reported that hepatic steatosis could be reversed following treatment with peroxisome proliferator-activated receptor alpha (PPAR-α) agonist which upregulated the enzymes involved in fatty acid β-oxidation.[16]

FATTY LIVER AND INSULIN RESISTANCE

Insulin resistance of hepatocytes are sufficient enough to induce hepatic steatosis. However, there are significant literature available that reports that the reverse is also viable, *i.e.*, hepatic steatosis can also induce hepatic insulin resistance.[17] Although the exact cellular and molecular mechanisms involved yet remains to be identified. It has been hypothesized that differences in lipid partitioning may be involved as the overexpression of malonyl coenzyme-A decarboxylase in the fatty hepatocytes of mice fed with high-fat diet induced hepatic steatosis decreases hepatic lipid accumulation and reverses fatty liver–associated hepatic, muscle, and systemic insulin resistance.[18]

Prevention of insulin resistance in mice with genetic- and/or diet-induced obesity through inhibition of stress-related protein kinase signaling cascade prevents insulin resistance.[19-20] These kinases has been reported to be a target for TNF-α activation[21]. In addition, inhibitor kappa beta kinase beta and p38 mitogen-activated protein kinase promotes the synthesis of TNF-α.[19,22] Thus, insulin resistance is both a consequence and a cause of increased TNF-α activity. However, in spite of the growing evidence that TNF-α could be a critical mediator of alcoholic steatohepatitis,[23] the possibility and feasibility that insulin resistance might play a key role in alcoholic steatohepatitis pathogenesis has not yet been explored. On the contrary, there are sufficient proof indicating the severity of insulin resistance with the severity of nonalcoholic steatohepatitis in humans.[24]

The human gastrointestinal tract homes approximately 10^{14} microorganisms, consisting mostly of commensals. Although, it primarily provides the host nutritional and energy needs along with shaping the host mucosal and systemic immunity, the gut microflora are increasingly recognized as an important pathogenic factor in chronic inflammation related diseases[25]. These physiological and pathological roles of gut microflora are mediated by following types of interactions: (1) inside the lumen of the gastrointestinal (GI) tract among microflora, or their metabolites, and different types of host cells at the surface of the intestinal epithelium; and (2) outside the GI tract between microbial products which have translocated across the intestinal epithelial barrier and the host cells in the circulation or in different organs.

The gut microflora florishes as a result of the rich environment provided by the availability of food. Normal flora thus prevent infections by competing for nutrients and binding sites thereby preventing pathogenic overgrowth.[26,27] Sometimes even commensal microbes that comprise the natural flora, can cause malabsorption, diarrhea, and infection. The mechanisms by which they induce the following includes (1) altered immune response, (2) translocation of bacteria due to increased intestinal permeability[28] and/or (3) simple alterations in the usual flora.[29] The human GI tract harbours an enormous number and variety of microorganisms, including atleast 10^{14} bacteria belonging to ~1,000 species[30]. The gut microbiota is predominantly comprising of species belonging to Firmicutes and Bacteroidetes, *i.e.*, with more than 90% population. The population are highly variable and diverse from person to person but having conserved set of core gut microbiota. The core microbiome are supposed to be common among individuals which may be necessary for gut functioning.[31-32] The Firmicutes are the largest phyla, with over 200 genera, including Mycoplasma, Lactobacillus, Clostridium and Bacillus species.[33]

It was first demonstrated in animal models for severe hemorrhagic shock co-associated with high mortality rate and with dietary hepatic injury that the role from a bacterial perspective in human diseases was identified as a causative agent even in the absence of a bacterial infection.[34] In these animal models, there were no apparent bacterial infection and the germ free animal models when given oral administration of non-absorbable antibiotics significantly improved the clinical outcomes. These germ-free animals were also resistant to diet induced liver injury.[35] The circulating endotoxin *i.e.*, Lipo Polysaccharides (LPS) had significantly elevated in these diseased animals, cound be a causative.[36] Further, when the antibiotic treated animals were given oral administration of LPS, it resensitized the animals to diet-induced liver injury conditions.[37] Recently, there are strong evidence which has indicated that translocation of microbial products and their role as a potential pathogenic inducers in a variety of chronic diseases such as chronic heart failure, spondyloarthritis, chronic fatigue syndrome, HIV/AIDS and AIDS-associated dementia, chronic hepatitis C, non-alcoholic steatohepatitis (as part of metabolic syndrome), and alcoholic liver disease to name a few.

LPS AND ALCOHOLIC FATTY LIVER

It has been clearly established in humans studies that heavy alcohol intake or consumption along with an increase in gut permeability and LPS leakage, may be associated with or without liver disease. Abstinence for 2 weeks or longer may be necessary for improving the gut permeability to return to its pre-alcoholic state.[38] A transient appreaence of LPS in the blood of normal human subjects has been observed following an Acute heavy alcohol consumption.[39] Individuals with alcoholic fatty liver but not severe liver disease also show an elevated LPS level in plasma.[40] Studies of animal models have shown that acute administration of alcohol in mice increased the LPS levels in plasma by five-fold within 30-90 min.[41-42] Daily binge feeding of alcohol in rats for 4 weeks increased the plasma LPS level approximately 15-fold compared to control animals.[43]

In addition to the adverse effect on gut barrier structure and permeability, chronic alcohol exposure also alters microflora content and composition. Alcoholics have an overgrowth of microflora in comparison to non-alcoholic individuals.[44] The overgrowth is predominantly seen in the Gram-negative bacteria *i.e.*, the LPS producing strains and thus increased its microbial products in the form of LPS in the gut and hence promoted their translocation. Chronic alcohol consumption also alters the composition of the microflora.[45] In line with these findings, when alcoholic animals and patients having alcoholic liver dieases were treated with probiotic or synbiotic administered, it restored the altered gut permeability and reduced tissue injury.[46]

Liver plays a key function in controlling the impact of microbial metabolies and products and thus becomes a critical factor during pathogenesis targeted at the liver. It has been shown in various clinical studies and experimental research that the liver plays a crucial role in the LPS clearance and inactivation. The mechanisms involved in reducing the LPS-induced inflammation in liver are: (1) the liver is known for its ability to detoxify and excrete LPS. Kupffer cells and hepatocytes are involved in detoxicifation of LPS while hepatocytes play an important role in its excretion (2) the excessive production of IL-10, an anti-inflammatory cytokines from the Kupffer cell's. The LPS which enters into the liver gets rapidly concentrated and then either they undergo hepatocytic degradation or undergo biliary excretion into the gut.[47,48] In a healthy liver, there is a rapid loss of biological activity of LPS,[49] whereas its spleenic uptake increases during the diseased state of liver.[48] Thus, the liver plays a primary and crucial role in protecting cells from exposure to microbial products.

Under compromised state of liver function, more microbial products enter and/or stay in circulation.[49] LPS tends to accumulate in other organs, such as spleen.[50,51] Consequently, the inflammatory response to the microbial products becomes exagerrated and prolonged. The impact of such circulating LPS on many organs might be significant, especially on the brain, and might exacerbate disease conditions in these organs.

ROLE OF TLRS DURING HEPATIC INFLAMMATION

Chronic liver disease (CLD) has been described as a state due to increased bacterial translocation which has triggered metabolic changes and/or viral infections. In patients with CLD, one of the major contributing factors for the defecin the intestinal mucosal barrier has altered intestinal motility. This alteration results in alteration of the intestinal microflora which contributes for decreased mucosal integrity, and suppressed immunity in CLD.[52] As a result of this breach in the intestinal barrier, there is an elevation in the circulating endotoxin levels which further triggers inflammation and fibrogenesis via Toll like receptors (TLR) signalling in the liver. TLRs are a family of pattern recognition receptors (PRRs) and function to maintain tissue homeostasis by regulating inflammatory responses and tissue repair.[53] Thirteen TLRs has been identified and structurally characterized by the presence of an individual leucine-rich repeat (LRR) domain in their extracellular domain and a Toll/IL-1 receptor (TIR) domain in their intracellular domain.[53] TLRs has been widely studied and TLR expression has been studies on Kupffer cells, endothelial cells, DCs, biliary epithelial cells, HSCs, and hepatocytes. TLRs thus may contribute to the progression of acute and chronic liver disease.

TLR4 has garnered much interest with respect to its role in hepatic inflammation and fibrogenesis[54]. In the liver, Kupffer cells have been known to be the foremost target for any bacterial attacks or sterile insults and to initiate any inflammatory responses. TLR4 expressed on the Kupffer cells has been involved in various liver diseases such as ischemia/reperfusion (I/R), alcohol-induced liver diseases, and diet-induced liver damages. LPS, ligand for TLR4, binds and results in the activaton of NF-kB, via various signalling pathways such as MAPK, ERK1, p38, JNK, and IRF3. This signalling cascade results in the production of proinflammatory cytokines and type I IFN, which enhance hepatocyte damage, increased leukocyte infiltration, and secretion of profibrogenic cytokines such a TGF-β and platelet-derived growth factor (PDGF), which in turn promotes the activation of hematopoietic stem cells (HSCs).[55]

Probiotics are live microbial dietary supplements which provides beneficial effects on host health.[56] Probiotics have attracted public attention because of their potential effectiveness for both the prevention and the treatment of immune diseases.[57] Probiotics have been knowingly ingested by humans for hundreds of years in the form of live yogurt. Probiotics have been used as growth promoters, for lactose intolerance, antitumour and anticholestrolaemic effects.[58]

Probiotic strains or consortium have been added to food items such as yogurt, dairy products (Lassi, ice cream), and are used in dietary supplements as tablet, capsule as well as in powder form. Probiotics should be able to withstand severe conditions of the stomach in the form of gastric acid and bile for the usefulness in the small and large intestine.[59] Among a wide range of probiotic strains, Lactobacilli and Bifidobacteria are the most widely used ones. Both these strains are gram-positive organisms that help produce lactic acid in order to remove harmful pathogens.[59]

Probiotic bacteria, usually administered at a concentration of 10^{8-9} cells, which colonize in the gut based on tolerance of gastric juice and small intestine. They colonize the gut for the short duration of time and disappear once the consumption stops. Lactobacillus or Bifidobacterium probiotic organisms can be recovered at a level ranging from 10^7 to 10^9 cells per gram corresponding to less than 0.1% of the fecal microbiota.[60] Scientific research has focused on how to use probiotic bacterial species such as Bifidobacteria and Lactobacilli to alter the composition of the indigenous gut microbiota.[61] These probiotic bacterial species help to protect the host by directly inhibiting the growth of harmful bacteria, and also benefit host health by reducing cholesterol levels, sustaining immune responses, and synthesizing vitamins such as folate and B12.[62]

Some of the most important representatives of lactobacilli are *L. acidophilus, L. casei, L. plantarum, L. crispatus, L. johnsonii, L. gallinarum, L. paracasei, L. reuteri, L. rhamnosus L. helveticus, L. gasseri, L. sake*, and from Bifidobacterium are *B. animalis, B. adolescentis, B. bifidum, B. breve, B. infantis, B. lactis and B. longum*. Other lactic acid bacteria such as *Enterococcus faecalis, E. faecium, Lactococcus lactis, Leuconostoc mesenteroides, Pediococcus acidilactis, Sporolactobacillus inulinus, Streptococcus thermophilus* and from non lactic acid bacteria such as *Bacillus cereus, Propionibacterium freudenreichii, Escherichia coli Nissle strain, Saccharomyces cerevisiae* and *S. boulardii* were generally used as probiotics.[63]

Various Lactobacillus strains has been used by different researcher for the management of diabetes and its complications with different mode of action for lowering blood glucose,[64] reducing the pancreatic and plasmatic α-amylase activities and level of plasma glucose,[65] improves insulin resistance and glucose intolerance,[66] decrease cholesterol levels and insulin sensitivity,[67] reduces blood lipid content,[68] improves gut colonization[69] and improves insulin resistance, glucose intolerance, oxidative stress, reduces IL-6 and TNF-α.[70]

Probiotics had been widely marketed and consumed, mostly as dietary supplements or functional foods. Mechanisms of probiosis include manipulation of intestinal microbial communities, suppression of pathogens, immunomodulation, stimulation of epithelial cell proliferation and differentiation and fortification of the intestinal barrier (Figure 2).[71] Probiotic strains induces an effect on composition and function of the intestinal microbiome. Probiotics produce antimicrobial agents or metabolic compounds that suppress the growth of other microorganisms,[72,73] or compete for receptors and binding sites with other intestinal microbes on the intestinal mucosa.[74] Probiotic Lactobacillus strains enhance the integrity of the intestinal barrier, which may result in maintenance of immune tolerance, decreased translocation of bacteria across the intestinal mucosa, and disease phenotypes such as gastrointestinal infections, IBS and IBD.[75] Moreover, probiotics can modulate the intestinal immunity and alter the responsiveness of the intestinal epithelia and immune cells to microbes in the intestinal lumen.[71,76]

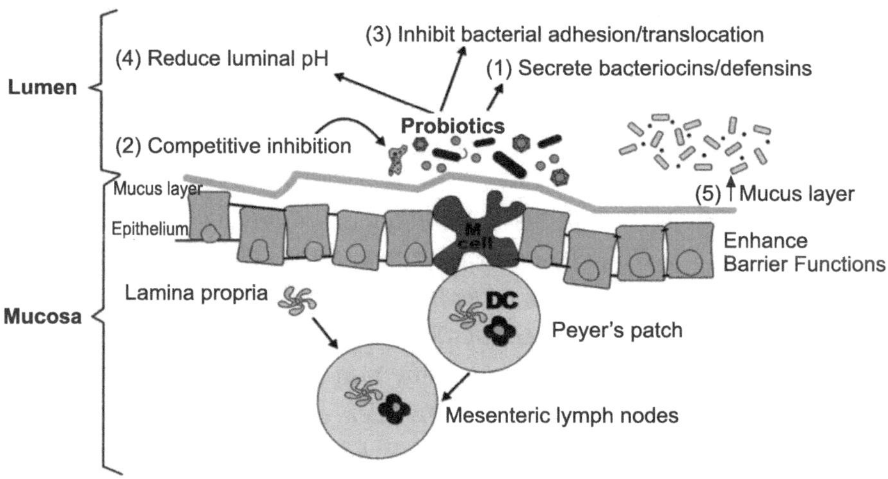

Fig. 2 Probiotic Mechanisms in the human gastrointestinal tract

The effects of probiotics on the composition, diversity and function of the gut microbiota have been studied using different tools and techniques ranging from targeted, culture-dependent methods to metagenomic sequencing. However, not many studies have demonstrated associations of altered microbiota following treatment with probiotics. A clinical study demonstrated decreased pain and flatulence in patients with IBS that received a 4-week treatment with a rose-hip drink containing 5×10^7 colony-forming units (CFU)/ml of *L. plantarum* DSM 9843 per day.[77] This improvement in clinical symptoms was associated with the presence of *L. plantarum* in rectal biopsies of patients, along with reduced amounts of enterococci in fecal specimens.

A more recent study focusing on patients with diarrhea- dominant IBS (IBS-D) yielded symptomatic relief in patients treated with a probiotic mixture of *L. acidophilus, L. plantarum, L. rhamnosus, Bifidobacterium breve, B. lactis, B. longum* and *Streptococcus thermophilus*.

PROBIOTIC TREATMENT STRATEGY IN LIVER DISEASES

The beneficial effects of probiotics on liver health were observed in several studies. The primary mechanisms reported in these studies are the changes in gut functions (Figure 3). Consumption of probiotics could allow enterobacteriaceae through the competitive inhibition. Developing nutritional practices, mucosal barrier repairing, apoptosis prevention due to providing of short chain acids, and improving intestinal epithelial viability are other probiotic effects which stabilize physiological luminal permeability together with lowering ammonia adsorption.[78] These functions alleviate tight junction disturbance by pathogens,[79] and are essential agents for lowering BT. Induction of anaerobes and gram positive bacteria growth, limiting gram negative bacteria, and preventing pathogens adherents are other anti-translocation effects of the probiotics.[80] Controlling flora bacteria quantity can lead to decreased endotoxins and other toxic compounds derived from bacteria such as ethanol, phenol, indoles which cause injury to the liver. Decreased levels of these substances in the liver result in lowering of proinflammatory production such as TNF-α, IL-6, and IFN-γ via down-regulation of the NF-κ B.[81] On the other hand, they can depress urease activity of microflora bacteria followed by ammonia production and release into the portal system. Furthermore, probiotic decreases fecal pH value and reduces ammonia adsorption.[82]

Although NAFLD is known as a prevalent type of liver disease globally, the preferred therapy method has not been established. To conquer the overpopulation of pathogens, antibiotic therapy is the current strategy. Polymixin B and metronidazole are antibiotics which are currently used in these patients for ameliorating liver functions. However, it is not an appropriate therapy because of the unspecific ramifications to any bacteria.[83] The usage of probiotic, prebiotic and symbiotic bacteria is recommended since these bacteria have the capacity to modulate microflora overpopulations and their consequent effect on the liver. In spite of the presence of various experimental studies in this field and positive effects of probiotic on induced liver steatosis, the recognition of this strategy for treating or even preventing NAFLD is still complicated. Furthermore, most of them were tested on animal models and insufficient human clinical trials have been performed. Therefore approving these bacteria as a treatment protocol requires several large scale clinical trials.

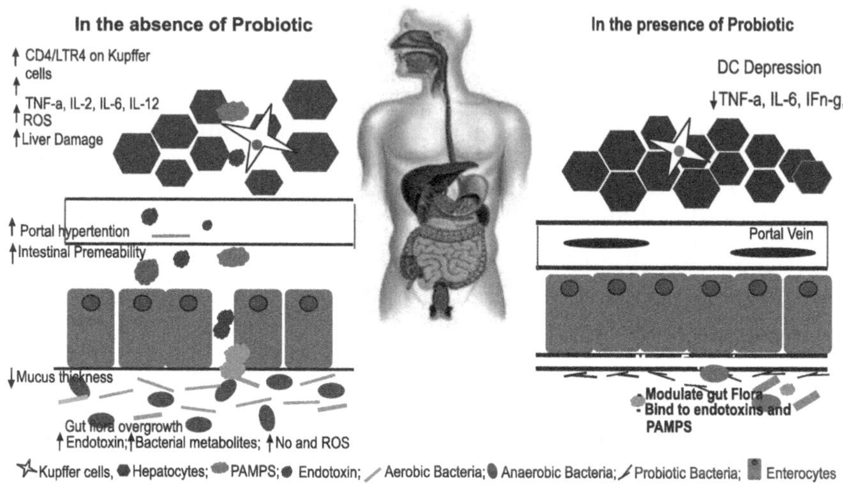

Fig. 3 Influence of Probiotic in Liver Disease

As such there is no optimal diet to treat NAFLD but experimental data showed role of probiotics on NAFLD and other inflammatory and metabolic disorder. High fructose diet (HFD) with fungal chitin-glucan (CG) showed decreased accumulation of hepatic triglyceride. CG treatment also reduces weight gain fat mass development, fasting hyperglycemia, glucose intolerance and hypercholesterolemia compared to HFD fed animals.[84] High fructose induced NAFLD mice when supplemented with *Lactobacillus rhamnosus* GG (LGC) showed reduction in liver fat accumulation, increased total numbers of Firmicutes and Bacteroidetes.[85,86]

Quantitative and qualitative alterations in the intestinal microflora are related to alcohol intake. In contrast to knowledge about most causative factors involved in the ALD pathogenesis, unfortunately, appropriate treatment of these patients is inconclusive as of yet. Since probiotic strains can modulate the gut and immune systems, it is suggested that probiotics can be administered to relieve ALD symptoms. Improving the liver variables such as serum liver enzyme (alanin aminotransferase, aspartate aminotransferase and gamma glutamyl transferase), and total bilirubin, ameliorating hepatic inflammation and histological grade are results from probiotic therapy in these studies.

Probiotics are found to suppress inflammatory condition by reducing serum LPS and expression of hepatic TNF-α. Probiotic also known to revert gut permeability. Lactobacillus species with or without arginine supplementation reduces translocation of bacteria[87] but lactobacillus fermented milk supplemented failed to reduce bacterial translocation in prehepatic portal hypertension experiments.[88,89] Gut microbiota modulation with certain antibiotics has been reported to decrease the liver inflammation in diet induced diabetes through TLR and NF-kB pathway.[90,91]

SUMMARY

A major instigate of liver disease is an anomaly in the gut flora. A balanced and healthy gut prevents a high percentage of harmful liver conditions. Several studies had been performed on various diseases, have confirmed the positive influence of probiotic strains on pathophysiological symptoms. Probiotic administration is safe, inexpensive and a noninvasive strategy as compared to antibiotic therapy and surgery. The expanding usage of antibiotics has resulted in the emergence of drug-resistant strains which pose a serious threat to humankind survival. Furthermore, the probiotic therapy shows no severe side effects unlike antibiotic therapy. Although results from clinical trials performed on common liver diseases showed the positive effects of probiotics, there are two problems that limit the usage of probiotics as a routine therapy. Since functional mechanisms of probiotic are specific to strain, recognize special strains with the highest prophylactic, and preventive properties on liver disease may be required. Also, engineering probiotics for specific, desirable properties might be useful.[92] Restoration or modulation of gut microflora has been recently taken a centre stage for inflammations associated with gastro-intestinal tract and its adjoining organs. Modulation using probiotics[93,94] or use of target specific antibiotic release encapsulated in microspheres needs to be further explored.[95] Lastly, to confirm the viability of bacteriotherapy, more clinical trials in various countries with disparate races, ethnicity, and lifestyles would be required.

ACKNOWLEDGMENTS

The author would like to acknowledge Nirma Education and Research Foundation, Ahmedabad for its financial support.

REFERENCES

1. C. Bode, J.C. BODE. Alcohol's Role in Gastrointestinal Tract Disorders. *Alcohol Health Res. W.* **1997**, 21 (1): 76-83.
2. P.S.S. Monga. Molecular Pathology of Liver Diseases, Springer US: Boston, MA, **2011.**
3. H. Tilg, A.M. Diehl. Cytokines in alcoholic and nonalcoholic steatohepatitis. *N. Engl. J. Med.* **2000**, 343: 1467–76.
4. R.G. Thurman. Mechanism of hepatic toxicity: II. Alcoholic liver injury involves activation of Kupffer cells by endotoxin. *Am. J. Physiol.* **1998**; 275: G605–11.
5. J.B. Hoek, P.G. Pastorino. Cellular signaling mechanisms in alcohol-induced liver damage. *Semin. Liver Dis.* **2004**; 24: 257–72.
6. B. Chassaing, L. Etienne-Mesmin, A.T. Gewirtz. Microbiota-liver axis in hepatic disease. *Hepatol.* **2014**, 59(1): 328-339.
7. E. Seki, B. Schnabl. Role of innate immunity and the microbiota in liver fibrosis: crosstalk between the liver and gut. *J. Physiol.* **2012**, 590: 447–458.
8. F.R. Ponziani, S. Pecere, A. Gasbarrini, V. Ojetti. Physiology and pathophysiology of liver lipid metabolism". *Expert Rev. Gastroenterol. Hepatol.* **2015**, 12: 1-13.
9. S. Sussman, C.W. Dent, S. Skara, P. de Calice, H. Tsukamoto. Alcoholic liver disease (ALD): a new domain for prevention efforts. *Subst. Use Misuse* **2002**, 37: 1887–1904.
10. S. Bellentani, G. Saccoccio, F. Masutti, L.S. Croce, G. Brandi, F. Sasso, G. Cristanini, C. Tiribelli. Prevalence of and risk factors for hepatic steatosis in Northern Italy. *Ann. Intern. Med.* **2000**, 132: 112–117.
11. S. Naveau, V. Giraud, E. Borotto, A. Aubert, F. Capron, J.C. Chaput. Excess weight risk factor for alcoholic liver disease. *Hepatol.* **1997**, 25: 108–111.

12. B. Raynard, A. Balian, D. Fallik, F. Capron, P. Bedossa, J.C. Chaput, S. Naveau. Risk factors of fibrosis in alcohol induced liver disease. *Hepatol.* **2002**, 35: 635–638.

13. C.J. Lyon, R.E. Law, W.A. Hsueh. Mini review: adiposity, inflammation, and atherogenesis. *Endocrinol.* **2003**, 144: 2195–2200.

14. S. Mora, J.E. Pessin. An adipocentric view of signaling and intracellular trafficking. *Diabetes Metab. Res. Rev.* **2002**, 18: 345–356.

15. K. Tobe, R. Suzuki, M. Aoyama *et.al.* Increased expression of the sterol regulatory element-binding protein-1 gene in insulin receptor substrate-2 / mouse liver. *J. Biol. Chem.* **2001**, 276: 38337–38340.

16. M. Fischer, M. You, M. Matsumoto, D.W. Crabb. Peroxisome proliferator-activated receptor (PPAR) agonist treatment reverses PPARg dysfunction and abnormalities in hepatic lipid metabolism in ethanol-fed mice. *J. Biol. Chem.* **2003**, 278: 27997–28004.

17. J.K. Kim, J.J. Fillmore, Y. Chen, C. Yu, I.K. Moore, M. Pypaert, E.P. Lutz, Y. Kako, W. Velez-Carrasco, I.J. Goldberg, J.L. Breslow, G.I. Shulman. Tissue-specific overexpression of lipoprotein lipase causes tissue-specific insulin resistance. *Proc. Natl. Acad. Sci. U.S.A.* **2001**, 98: 7522–7527.

18. J. An, D.M. Muoio, M. Shiota et. al. Hepatic expression of malonyl-CoA decarboxylase reverses muscle, liver and whole-animal insulin resistance. *Nat. Med.* **2004**, 10: 268–274.

19. R.J. Gum, L.L. Gaede, M.A. Heindel *et.al.* Antisense protein tyrosine phosphatase 1B reverses activation of p38 mitogen-activated protein kinase in liver of ob/ob mice. *Mol. Endocrinol.* **2003**, 17: 1131–1143.

20. J. Hirosumi, G. Tuncman, L. Chang, C.Z. Go¨rgu¨n, K.T. Uysal, K. Maeda, M. Karin, G.S. Hotamisligil. A central role for JNK in obesity and insulin resistance. *Nature* **2002**, 420: 333–336.

21. H. Wajant, K. Pfizenmaier, P. Scheurich. Tumor necrosis factor signaling. *Cell Death Differ*. **2003**, 10: 45–65.

22. N. Sizemore, N. Lerner, N. Dombrowski, H. Sakurai, G.R. Stark. Distinct roles of the IkB kinase a and b subunits in liberating nuclear factor kB (NF-kB) from IkB and in phosphorylating the p65 subunit of NF-kB. *J. Biol. Chem.* **2002**, 277: 3863–3869.

23. H. Tsukamoto, S.C. Lu. Current concepts in the pathogenesis of alcoholic liver injury. *FASEB J.* **2001**, 15: 1335–1349.

24. G. Marchesini, E. Bugianesi, G. Forlani *et.al.* Nonalcoholic fatty liver, steatohepatitis, and the metabolic syndrome. *Hepatol*. **2003**, 37: 917–923.

25. D. Artis. Epithelial-cell recognition of commensal bacteria and maintenance of immune homeostasis in the gut. *Nat. Rev. Immunol*. **2008**, 8: 411-420.

26. U. Vyas, N. Ranganathan. Probiotics, prebiotics, and synbiotics: gut and beyond. *Gastroenterol. Res. Prac.* **2012**; 872716.

27. T. Murguía-Peniche, W.A. Mihatsch, J. Zegarra, S. Supapannachart, Z.Y. Ding, J. Neu. Intestinal mucosal defense system, Part 2. Probiotics and prebiotics. *J. Pediatr.* **2013**, 162: 64-71.

28. S. Elavarasu, P. Jayapalan, T. Murugan. Bugs that debugs: Probiotics. *J. Pharm. Bioall. Sci.* **2012**, 4: 319-22.

29. B. Kligler, A. Cohrssen. Probiotics. *Am. J. Fam. Physician* **2008**, 78(9): 1073-78.

30. A.S. Neish, A.T. Gewirtz, H. Zeng, A.N. Young, M.E. Hobert, V. Karmali, A.S. Rao, J.L. Madara. Prokaryotic regulation of epithelial responses by inhibition of IkB-a ubiquitination. *Science* **2000**, 289: 1560-1563.

31. P.J. Turnbaugh, V.K. Ridaura, J.J. Faith, F.E. Rey, R. Knight, J.I. Gordon. The effect of diet on the human gut microbiome: a metagenomic analysis in humanized gnotobiotic mice. *Sci. Transl. Med.* **2009**, 1: 6- 14.

32. J. Qin, R. Li, J. Raes *et.al.* A human gut microbial gene catalogue established by metagenomic sequencing. *Nature* **2010**; 464: 59–65.

33. E.G. Zoetendal, A.D. Akkermans, W.M. De Vos. Temperature gradient gel electrophoresis analysis of 16S rRNA from human fecal samples reveals stable and host-specific communities of active bacteria. *Appl. Environ. Microbiol.* **1998**, 64: 3854-9.

34. J. Fine, H. Frank, F. Schweinburg, S. Jacob, T. Gordon. The bacterial factor in traumatic shock. *Ann. N. Y. Acad. Sci* **1952**, 55, 429-445.

35. T.D. Luckey, J.A. Reyniers, P. Gyorgy, M. Forbes. Germ-free animals and liver necrosis. *Ann. N. Y. Acad. Sci.* **1954**, 57, 932-935.

36. H.A. Ravin, D. Rowley, C. Jenkins, J. Fine. On the absorption of bacterial endotoxin from the gastro-intestinal tract of the normal and shocked animal. *J. Exp. Med.* **1960**, 112, 783-792.

37. S.A. Broitman, L.S. Gottlieb, N. Zamcheck. Influence of neomycin and ingested endotoxin in the pathogenesis of choline deficiency cirrhosis in the adult rat. *J. Exp. Med.* **1964**, 119, 633-642.

38. I. Bjarnason, T.J. Peters, R.J. Wise. The leaky gut of alcoholism: possible route of entry for toxic compounds. *Lancet* **1984**, 1, 179-182.

39. C. Bode, V. Kugler, J.C. Bode. Endotoxemia in patients with alcoholic and non-alcoholic cirrhosis and in subjects with no evidence of chronic liver disease following acute alcohol excess. *J. Hepatol.* **1987**, 4, 8-14.

40. H. Fukui, B. Brauner, J.C. Bode, C. Bode. Plasma endotoxin concentrations in patients with alcoholic and non-alcoholic liver disease: reevaluation with an improved chromogenic assay. *J. Hepatol. 1991*, 12, 162-169

41. C.A. Rivera, B.U. Bradford, V. Seabra, R.G. Thurman. Role of endotoxin in the hypermetabolic state after acute ethanol exposure. *Am. J. Physiol.* **1998**, 275, G1252-G1258.

42. Z. Zhou, L. Wang, Z. Song, J.C. Lambert, C.J. McClain, Y.J. Kang. A critical involvement of oxidative stress in acute alcohol induced hepatic TNF-alpha production. *Am. J. Pathol.* **2003**, 163, 1137-1146.

43. N. Enomoto, S. Yamashina, H. Kono *et.al.* Development of a new, simple rat model of early alcohol-induced liver injury based on sensitization of Kupffer cells. *Hepatol.* **1999**, 29, 1680-1689.

44. J.C. Bode, C. Bode, R. Heidelbach, H.K. Dürr, G.A. Martini. Jejunal microflora in patients with chronic alcohol abuse. *Hepato-gastroenterol.* **1984**, 31, 30-34.

45. T. Hauge, J. Persson, D. Danielsson. Mucosal bacterial growth in the upper gastrointestinal tract in alcoholics (heavy drinkers). *Dig.* **1997**, 58, 591-595.

46. I.A. Kirpich, N.V. Solovieva, S.N. Leikhter, N.A. Shidakova, O.V. Lebedeva, P.I. Sidorov, T.A. Bazhukova, A.G. Soloviev, S.S. Barve, C.J. McClain, M. Cave. Probiotics restore bowel flora and improve liver enzymes in human alcohol-induced liver injury: a pilot study. *Alcohol* **2008**, 42, 675-682.

47. Y. Mimura, S. Sakisaka, M. Harada, M. Sata, K. Tanikawa. Role of hepatocytes in direct clearance of lipopolysaccharide in rats. *Gastroenterol.* **1995**, 109, 1969-1976.

48. Y. Nakatani, H. Fukui, H. Kitano *et.al.* Endotoxin clearance and its relation to hepatic and renal disturbances in rats with liver cirrhosis. *Liver* **2001**, 21: 64-70.

49. A. Sandek, S.D. Anker, S. von Haehling. The gut and intestinal bacteria in chronic heart failure. *Curr. Drug Metab.* **2009**, 10: 22-28.

50. G. Tachiyama, M. Sakon, J. Kambayashi, S. Iijima, T. Tsujinaka, T. Mori. Endogenous endotoxemia in patients with liver cirrhosis--a quantitative analysis of endotoxin in portal and peripheral blood. *Jpn. J. Surg.* **1988**, 18: 403-408.

51. M. Freudenberg, C. Galanos. Metabolic fate of endotoxin in rat. *Adv. Exp. Med. Biol.* **1990**, 256, 499-509.

52. O. Takeuchi, S. Akira. Pattern recognition receptors and inflammation. Cell 2010, 140, 805–820.

53. E. Seki, B. Schnabl. Role of innate immunity and the microbiota in liver fibrosis: crosstalk between the liver and gut. *J. Physiol.* **2012**, 590, 447–458.

54. E. Seki, D.A. Brenner. Toll-like receptors and adaptor molecules in liver disease: update. *Hepatol.* **2008**, 48, 322–335.

55. T. Aoyama, P. Yong-Han, S. Ekihiro. Toll-like receptor signaling and liver fibrosis. *Gastroenterol. Res. Pract.* **2010**, http://dx.doi.org/10.1155/2010/192543.

56. FAO/WHO. Health and nutritional properties and guidelines for evaluation of Probiotic in foods. *FAO Food Nutr. Pap.* **2006**, 85, ISBN 92-5-105513-0

57. A.T. Borchers, C. Selmi, F.J. Meyers, C.L. Keen, M.E. Gershwin. Probiotics and immunity. *J. Gastroenterol.* **2009,** 44: 26-46.

58. H. Singh, H. Singh. Probiotics – An Emerging Concept. *Int. J. Sci. Res. Pub.* **2014**, 4(6): 1-3.

59. T.R. Klaenhammer, M.J. Kullen. Selection and design of probiotics. *Int.J. Food Microbiol.* **1999**, 50: 45-57.

60. Ruth E. Ley, Fredrik Bäckhed, Peter Turnbaugh, Catherine A. Lozupone, Robin D. Knight and Jeffrey I. Gordon. Obesity alters gut microbial ecology. *Proc. Nat. Acad. Sci.* **2005**, 102: 11070-5.

61. G.R. Gibson, C.M. Williams Eds. Functional Foods: Concept to Product (Woodhead Publishing, CRC Press) **2000**, 85-88

62. S. Khani, H.M. Hosseini, M. Taheri, M.R. Nourani, F.A.A. Imani. Probiotics as an alternative strategy for prevention and treatment of human diseases: a review. *Inflamm. Allergy Drug Targets* **2012**, 11: 79-89.

63. M. Kechagia, D. Basoulis, S. Konstantopoulou, D. Dimitriadi, K. Gyftopoulou, N. Skarmoutsou, E.M. Fakiri. Health benefits of probiotics: a review. *ISRN Nutrition* **2013**; 481651.

64. J.H. Yun, K.B. Lee, Y.K. Sung, E.B. Kim, H.G. Lee, Y.J. Choi. Isolation and Characterization of potential probiotic lactobacilli from pig feces. *J. Basic Microbiol.* **2009**, 49: 220-226.

65. W. Bejar, K. Hamden, B.R. Salah, H. Chouayekh. Bacillus plantarum TN627 significantly reduces complications of alloxan-induced diabetes in rats. *Anaerobe* **2013**, 24: 4-11

66. N.J. Tripolt, B. Leber, D. Blattl *et.al.* Effect of supplementation with Lactobacillus casei Shirota on insulin sensitivity, beta-cell function, and markers of endothelial function and inflammation in subjects with metabolic syndrome--a pilot study. *J. Dairy Sci.* **2013**, 96: 89-95.

67. M. Kumar, S. Rakesh, R. Nagpal *et.al.* Probiotic Lactobacillus rhamnosus GG and Aloe vera gel improve lipid profiles in hypercholesterolemic rats. *Nutrition* **2013**, 29(3), 574–579.

68. H. Yadav, S. Jain, P.R. Sinha. Antidiabetic effect of probiotic dahi containing Lactobacillus acidophilus and Lactobacillus casei in high fructose fed rats. *Nutrition* **2006**; 23(1): 62-68.

69. R. Teanpaisan, J. Hintao, G. Dahlén. Oral Lactobacillus species in type 2 diabetic patients living in southern Thailand. *Anaerobe* **2009**, 15: 160-3.

70. F.G. Hsieh, C.L. Lee, C.Y Chai, W.T. Chen, Y.C. Lu, C.S. Wu. Oral administration of Lactobacillus reuteri GMNL-263 improves insulin resistance and ameliorates hepatic steatosis in high fructose-fed rats. *Nutr. Metab.* **2013**, 10: 35.

71. C. Thomas, J. Versalovic. Probiotics-host communication: modulation of signaling pathways in the intestine. *Gut Microbes* **2010**, 1, 148–163.

72. J. Spinler, M. Taweechotipatr, C. Rognerud, C. Ou, S. Tumwasorn, J. Versalovic. Human derived probiotic Lactobacillus reuteri demonstrate antimicrobial activities targeting diverse enteric bacterial pathogens. *Anaerobe* **2008**, 14, 166–171.

73. E. O'Shea, P. Cotter, C. Stanton, R. Ross, C. Hill. Production of bioactive substances by intestinal bacteria as a basis for explaining probiotic mechanisms: bacteriocins and conjugated linoleic acid. *Int. J. Food Microbiol.* **2011**, 152, 189–205.

74. M. Collado, J. Meriluoto, S. Salminen. Role of commercial probiotic strains against human pathogen adhesion to intestinal mucus. *Lett. Appl. Microbiol.* **2007**, 45, 454–460.

75. B. Lee, Y. Bak. Irritable bowel syndrome, gut microbiota and probiotics. *J. Neurogastroenterol. Motil.* **2011**, 17, 252–266.

76. P. Bron, P. Van Baarlen, M. Kleerebezem. Emerging molecular insights into the interaction between probiotics and the host intestinal mucosa. *Nat. Rev. Microbiol.* **2011**, 10, 66–78.

77. S. Nobaek, M. Johansson, G. Molin, S. Ahrne, B. Jeppsson. Alteration of intestinal microflora is associated with reduction in abdominal bloating and pain in patients with irritable bowel syndrome. *Am. J. Gastroenterol.* **2000**, 95, 1231–1238.

78. O. Kanauchi, Y. Fujiyama, K. Mitsuyama *et. al.* Increased growth of Bifidobacterium and Eubacterium by germinated barley foodstuff, accompanied by enhanced butyrate production in healthy volunteers. *Int. J. Mol. Med.* **1999**, 3(2), 175- 9.

79. K.C. Johnson-Henry, K.A. Donato, G. Shen-Tu, M. Gordanpour, P.M. Sherman. Lactobacillus rhamnosus strain GG prevents enterohemorrhagic Escherichia coli O157:H7-induced changes in epithelial barrier function. *Infect. Immun.* **2008**, 76(4), 1340-8.

80. H.Y. Zhao, H.J. Wang, Z. Lu, S.Z. Xu. Intestinal microflora in patients with liver cirrhosis. *Chin. J. Dig. Dis.* **2004**, 5(2), 64-7.

81. D.J. O'Sullivan. Genomics can advance the potential for probiotic cultures to improve liver and overall health. *Curr. Pharm. Des.* **2008**, 14(14), 1376-81.

82. M.R. Clausen, P.B. Mortensen. Lactulose, disaccharides and colonic flora. Clinical consequences. *Drugs* **1997**, 53(6), 930-42.

83. L. Miele, V. Valenza, G. La Torre *et.al.* Increased intestinal permeability and tight junction alterations in nonalcoholic fatty liver disease. *Hepatol.* **2009**, 49(6), 1877-87.

84. A.M. Neyrinck, S. Possemiers, W. Verstraete, F. Backer, P.D. Cani, N.M. Delzenne. Dietary modulation of clostridial cluster XIV a gut bacteria (Roseburia spp.) by chitin-glucan fiber improves host metabolic alterations induced by high-fat diet in mice. *J. Nutr. Biochem.* **2012**, 23(1), 51– 59.

85. Y. Ritze, G. Bárdos, A. Claus, V. Ehrmann, I. Bergheim, A. Schwiertz, S.C. Bischoff . Lactobacillus rhamnosus GG protects against non-alcoholic fatty liver disease in mice. *PLoS ONE* **2014**, 9(1), e80169.

86. E. Lau, D. Carvalho, P. Freitas. Gut Microbiota: Association with NAFLD and Metabolic Disturbances. *BioMed. Res. Int.* **2015**, 2015, 979515.

87. D. Adawi, F.B. Kasravi, G. Molin, B. Jeppsson. Effect of Lactobacillus supple- mentation with and without arginine on liver damage and bacterial translocation in an acute liver injury model in the rat. *Hepatol.* **1997**, 25, 642–647.

88. R. Wiest, F. Chen, G. Cadelina, R.J. Groszmann, G. Garcia-Tsao. Effect of Lactobacillus-fermented diets on bacterial translocation and intestinal flora in experimental prehepatic portal hypertension. *Dig. Dis. Sci.* **2003**, 48, 1136–1141.

89. E.M.M. Quigley, C. Stanton, E.F. Murphy. The Gut Microbiota and the Liver. Pathophysiological and Clinical Implications. *J. Hepatol.* **2013**, 58(5), 1020–27.

90. B. Prajapati, J.K. Jena, P. Rajput, K. Purandhar, S. Seshadri. Understanding and modulating the Toll like Receptors (TLRs) and NOD like Receptors (NLRs) Cross Talk in Type 2 Diabetes. *Curr. Diabetes Rev.* **2014**, 3(10), 190-200.

91. B. Prajapati, J.K. Jena, P. Rajput, S. Seshadri. Role of Pattern Recognition Receptors and inflammatory mediators following gut microbiota alteration in high sugar diet mediated type 2 diabetes". *J. Obesity Weight Loss Ther.* **2014**, 4(5), S1-014.

92. D. Trivedi, P.K. Jena, S. Seshadri. Colicin E2 Expression in Lactobacillus brevis DT24. A vaginal probiotic isolates against Uropathogenic Escherichia coli. *ISRN Urology* **2014**, 2014: 869610.

93. P.K. Jena, S. Singh, B. Prajapati, G. Nareshkumar, T. Mehta, S. Seshadri, Impact of Targeted Specific Antibiotic Delivery for Gut Microbiota Modulation on High Fructose Fed Rats. *Appl. Biochem. Biotechnol.* **2014,** 172, 3810-3826.

94. P.K. Jena, S. Singh, B. Prajapati, P.K. Mishra, S. Seshadri. Influence of Gut Microbiota on Inflammation and Pathogenesis of Sugar Rich diet induced Diabetes. *Immunome Res.* **2016**, 12(1): 109-119.

95. P. Bhumika, P. Rajput, P.K. Jena, S. Seshadri. Investigation of Chitosan for Prevention of Diabetic Progression through Gut Microbiota alteration in sugar rich diet induced diabetic rats. *Curr. Pharm. Biotechnol.* **2016**, 17: 173-184.

Editors' Note

Prolonged use of alcohol increases the risks of chronic liver disease, fatty liver disease, Fibrosis, Cirrhosis, Alcoholic hepatitis etc. Since, liver controls detoxification, absorption of nutrients and digestion of food. Hence, probiotics for liver health is suggested as an alternative to the use of antibiotics. Probiotics helps in intestinal immunity and also in epithelial viability. Probiotics are beneficial also in improving overall health and hence used as nutritional supplements. The damage to liver with the use of probiotics can be minimized.

❑❑❑

7

Herbal and Natural Medicines for Treatment of Alcoholism and Associated Diseases

Jyoti Singh

Abstract

Alcohol consumption is a severe addiction problem that leads to a number of health and social issues. Various herbs and plant based formulations have been reported for the de-addiction of alcoholic persons and also for the treatment of various ailments associated with heavy drinking particularly the liver diseases. In this chapter, natural therapies, various herbs and plants formulations that have beneficial effects for treatment of alcoholic person for de-addiction and alcoholism associated diseases have been discussed.

Keywords: Herbal medicine, Phytopharmaceuticals, Alcoholism, Liver disease

INTRODUCTION

Alcohol consumption is known to be a very old practice, its origin could be nearly as old as can be associated with the development of human civilizations in ancient time. The alcohol consumption vary from person to person, in early stages small amount of alcohol (the ethyl alcohol) would be sufficient to bring its alcohol induced eccentric effects while with passage

* Department of Botany, M.K.J.K. Mahavidyalaya, M.D. University, Rohtak, Haryana 124001. India.

of time a larger amount would be required to bring the same level of effect in the same person. Generally, person start consuming large amount of alcohol with passage of time and also the frequency of drinking enhances. This frequent heavy drinking is called 'Alcohol Addiction' or 'Alcoholic' stage.[1]

The various stages of alcohol drinking from beginner to alcohol addiction could be defined in following types[2]:

1. **Adaptive stage or Beginner stage:** It is the early stage of starting or testing alcoholic drinks. Person believes that he/she can tolerate it. Initially, a small quantity would be sufficient to bring effect of alcohol on person. Gradually the quantity of consumption increases. This is a non noticeable stage.
2. **Progressive Stage:** The person is able to tolerate larger amount of alcohol compared to beginners. The person would start and tend to consume large amount of alcohol though may be infrequent in consumption.
3. **Dependence stage:** In this stage person needs a large quantity than the earlier, the person becomes dependent to alcohol for performing daily activities. He/she becomes addict. To avoid withdrawal the person further increases consumption.
4. **Deterioration stage:** At this stage the alcohol consumption starts affecting badly or damaging various body organs, and patient gets mental disorder. This is heavy drinking stage, the person would drink any time in the day or night. The body organs get affected badly, the person could be abusive, not able to walk properly or control the body.

Habit Level Stages

1. **Planned drinker:** Person plans carefully when and how to take drink. He drinks on particular occasions like Birthday, Festivals, Promotion, Marriage anniversary etc. During other times, he abstains himself from alcohol.
2. **Bridge drinker:** Person drinks through a day time in unlimited manner, for a specific period of a week or two weeks. After that he stops drinking. It is a transit stage in between planned drinking and daily drinking.

3. **Daily drinker:** These persons drinks throughout the day. There is no fixed pattern of drinking and frequency of drinking. The daily drinkers even keep a bottle near to their bed. These are categorically the heavy drinkers.

In mild amounts, the ethyl alcohol have beneficial medical effects (it has antibiotic properties) such as treatment of sore throats or coughing,[3] however, large amount or frequent drinking of ethyl alcohol create health complications. Many chronic diseases and nutritional deficiencies are associated with alcohol consumption patterns such as average volume of alcohol consumed, quality of the alcoholic beverages consumed, as well as age, health and sex of the consumer. Alcoholism or alcohol addiction results in medical complications, and generate social and economic problems throughout the world. The alcohol affects entire human body and excessive consumption of alcohol generally induces unpleasant physical symptoms such as headache, nausea and vomiting in non drinkers. Even in regular drinkers, consumption of large quantities of alcohol at one time might induce acute alcohol toxicity with acidosis, heart failure and respiratory depression caused by an autonomic nerve and cerebrum dysfunction. Person consuming alcohol in large doses start losing control over body and respond time to any stimuli also get increased. Further, continuous consumption of alcohol over long time in large quantities induces a number of health disorders such as liver diseases (fatty liver, alcoholic hepatitis, hepatocirrhosis), gastrointestinal disorder, digestive problems, chronic pancreatitis, peripheral nervous disorder (losing control over limb movements), myocardosis, hypertension and haematopoiesis disorders. As alcoholism affect decision making capacity and nervous system of a person, the long-term alcohol consumption also causes mental illness which causes drastic change in behaviour toward family, friends & colleagues which further consequent into social effects, such as violent crimes and traffic accidents.

The treatment for alcoholism would mean to reduce the desire for alcohol, as well to combat the withdrawal symptoms alongwith, treating the side effects or damaged organs including psychological mental stabilization of the patient. Any treatment for alcohol deaddication would be a comprehensive therapy with consideration of different aspects and combination of different therapies. The single molecular or chemical therapy prove insufficient, with many side effects at most times. The traditional natural therapies supplemented with herbal medicines would be more promising in reducing the withdrawal symptoms and better recovery of patient.

In modern medicine (allopathy), the molecular receptors are targeted by different chemical drugs for treatment of alcoholism. The chemical drugs and targets for treatment of alcoholism include benzodiazepines, complex vitamins, cyanamide disulfiram and aldehyde dehydrogenase inhibitors. These chemical drugs are administered to alcoholic patients to suppress withdrawal symptoms and decrease appetite for drinking. However, as is the case with most of the chemical drugs, most of these chemical drugs have side effects and generally lead to abuse, psychological dependence and adverse behavioural effects. Many of drugs used for treatment of alcoholism could also lead to physiological dependence when taken chronically (as these are meant for closure of targets and patient body adapts to doses of drugs), and this ultimately results in dose escalation. Aldehydedehydrogenase inhibitors, especially disulfiram, have been reported to show serious side effects. The drug naltrexone, an opioid receptor antagonist, is being used for treating alcoholism in humans. Although naltrexone suppresses alcohol consumption, it has some side effects, including the development of withdrawal symptoms, nausea, dysphoria and fatigue. Another drug acamprosate (campral), approved by the US Food and Drug Administration (FDA) for alcoholism treatment, has been demonstrated to be safe and effective by multiple clinical studies involving alcohol-dependent people, its efficacy and mechanisms are not fully understood. The most common side effects reported for patients taking campral in clinical trials include headache, diarrhoea, flatulence and nausea.

In lieu of large number of side effects of chemical drugs, alternative therapies and medicines have been used for the treatment of alcoholism. Many alternative medicines were used even before the discovery of the synthetic chemical drugs, and were in practice in many countries particularly Asian countries. Many traditional medicines and natural products have been known to have preventive and therapeutic effects for alcoholism. Further, combination of concepts of modern medicine with the traditional therapies have produced better pharmaceutics for different ailments. The exploration of experimental evidence and re-examination of empirical data from traditional medicines (including chemical exploration of natural products) has opened new avenue, provided the lead towards novel pharmacological approaches for the treatment of alcoholism along with the application of alternative therapies. In this chapter, we have discussed different selected alternative natural therapies, their fundamental concepts of applications, research progress on natural therapies and herbal medicines for the treatment of alcoholism, and herbal drugs used for treatment of alcoholism associated diseases particularly the liver infections.

AYURVEDIC CONCEPT OF ALCOHOLISM

Ayurveda, the ancient Indian traditional health care system (ayus-life, veda-knowledge, meaning science of life), is the oldest medical system in the world and has been the prominent treatment therapy in the Indian region. The Ayurveda provides an integrated approach to prevention and treatment of different diseases by a large number of medical procedures and plants based pharmaceuticals. One of the clinical approaches of Ayurveda is Rasayana. Rasayana is not only a drug therapy but also a specialized procedure practiced through rejuvenating recipes in a dietary regimen promoting good habits. The purpose of rasayana is optimization of homeostasis in order to prevent disease and also cure different ailments. The meaning of the word Rasayana (rasa-essence, water; ayana-going) essentially refers to nutrition and its acquisition and circulation in the body tissues. Ayurveda treats the patients by balancing the three components *Vaat*, *Pitt*, and *Kaff* in the body. It cures the patients by providing supplements for balancing all the three components through herbal extracts and/or body exercises.[4]

Ayurveda considers the consumption of large quantities of alcohol as *Visha* – toxic. In Ayurveda, the alcohol itself is defined by its various *gunas* (properties) which help in understanding its impact on the human body and also in designing the treatment.

Properties of alcohol as per Ayurveda: As described in the Ayurvedic texts alcohol has following properties.[5] *Laghu* (light, small), *Ushna* (hot), *Tikshna (*sharp), *Visada* (drying), *Vikaasa* (expensive), *Ruksha* (rough), *Aasuga* (swift), *Vyavyal* (prevador), *Amla* (sour), *Sookshma (*subtle). These defined properties of alcohol helps in understanding its impact on the body.

The Ayurveda treatment for alcoholism work on different angles simultaneously to provide the comprehensive treatment to the patients. The therapy concentrates and includes the clearing of alcohol from body by different procedure and body exercises, reduction of desire and combating withdrawal symptoms by using various herbal extracts/medicines, giving supplemental ayurvedic medicines for controlling the damaged organs or for healthy working of affected organs, and meditation which help in increasing the confidence and self-controlling the desire to consume alcohol. These aspects and herbal medicines used in ayurveda for treatment of alcoholism are explained in following paragraphs.

AYURVEDIC TREATMENT FOR ALCOHOLISM

The Ayurveda being a comprehensive treatment, it emphasize to bring the patient body to the normal state. The first part of treatment include the detoxification of body *i.e.* clearing of alcohol and other toxics from body of alcoholic person.[6]

The alcoholic person is given Panchakarma treatment[7] in the beginning. Panchakarma (Panch – five, karma – actions) is a set of five therapies designed mainly for cleansing the body of toxins.[7] Ayurveda considers that the purification of the body is important before the commencement of any other therapy. It helps the body to normal functioning state of organs. The panchkarma involve following therapies (these must be performed in guidance of an expert in beginning):[8,9]

Vamana – vomiting therapy:

The Vamana is physical activity in which a patient has to drink large amount of warm salted water (sometime herbal extracts may also be added components) and then has to vomit the whole drinked water (forced vomiting by tickling the vulva area with fingers) in bent position of the body. This is meant to clean the stomach. This is given to people with high Kapha imbalance. Daily treatment involves loosening and mobilizing the toxins in an effort to finally eliminate them. After completing this exercise, patient must not drink water (particularly cold or normal temperature water) and must not take bath for atleast 1 hour after this.[6]

Virechana – purgative therapy

It is the procedure of taking warm water in excess and cleaning the whole intestine/digestive system. It completely cleanses the gastro-intestinal tract. The person has to avoid taking bath in cold weather on the day purgative is done. This must be preformed in presence and guidance of an expert.[8]

Basti – enema therapy

In this therapy, the rectum of patient is filled with salted water through anus and then passed out after sometime. This help in cleansing the rectum.

Medicated oil or ghee and an herbal decoction may also be given as enema to clean the colon and increase the muscle tone. This treatment is provided for several days, based on the medical condition of a person.

Nasya – nasal drops therapy

In nasya panchkarma exercise, the water or ghee is administered from one nostril and brought out from other nostril. It cleans the nostrils and throat.

Panchkarma Diet

A controlled diet is must on the days of the above Panchakarma practices/ exercise are performed. Panchkarma is effective only if simple prescribed food is taken or special detoxification diet is consumed along with the treatments.

The Panchkarma detoxifies body and mind and prepares the body for oral medication and other further treatments.

IMPORTANT AYURVEDIC HERBS USED IN THE TREATMENT OF ALCOHOLISM

There are a number of herbs formulations (prepared by thorough processing) which are used in Ayurveda to reduce the desire to take alcoholic beverages, control the withdrwal symptoms, bringing the affected organs to normal functions. Generally, these herbal formulations are given in combinations which provide dual or multiple benefits to patients. The amount of herbs given is generally low for slow actions; though by this therapy is longered but this reduces the side effects.

In following sections, the herbs used in ayurveda are mentioned along with their main impacts and also evaluations of respective herbs by modern experimentations, if any.

Herbs to Improve Memory, Concentration and to Fight Depression

Mental control and strength is essential for any alcoholic person in generating the confidence and stamina for alcoholism treatment. The following herbs are used for increasing the memory, and most of it is used as brain tonic to increase concentration. These, in general, help in fighting alcoholism associated depression.

Shankhpushpi (*Convolvulus pluricaulis*)

Shankhpushpi (*Convolvulus pluricaulis*) (Figure 1) have characteristic trumpet shaped flowers and is known as ethnopharmacologically, a brain tonic with anti-anxiety, anticonvulsant, anti-depressant and nootropic properties. The Shankhpushpi churna (powder) have been reported to reduce the alcohol withdrawal anxiety in a dose-dependent manner. The shankhpushpi was tested on the mice fed with alcohol for 21 days. The treatment using shankhpushpi decreased ethanol intake and increased water intake significantly after 4 days administration. These effects of alcohol reduction and further increased water intake were blocked by $GABA_A$ antagonists which suggested the involvement of $GABA_A$ receptors in de-addiction process (the expected target for shankpushpi by general end effects). Further, chronic administration of shankhpushpi also significantly increased cortico-hippocampal GABA level in mice. Shankhpushpi, thus, reduced both alcohol dependence and withdrawal symptoms of alcoholism by acting on and involvement of $GABA_A$receptors. Shankpushpi, thus, have been shown to possess anti-addictive potential for alcoholism.[10]

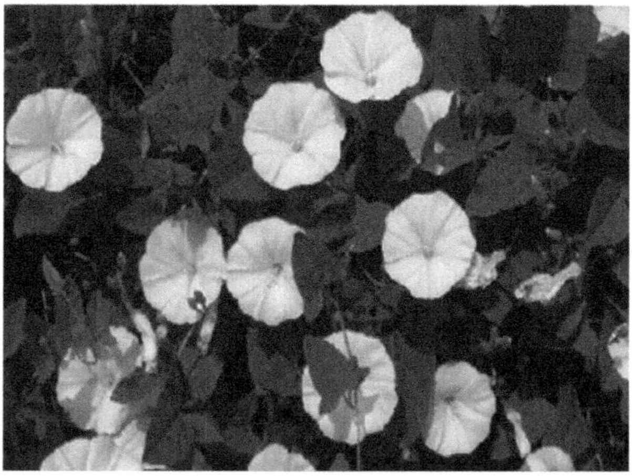

Fig. 1 Plant of Shankhpushpi (*Convolvulus pluricaulis*). Source: Google images.

Kanphool - Dandeleon/Dandelion (*Taxacum officinale*)

The Kanphool or Dandelion (Figure 2) is a popular herb in ayurveda, known to have high medicinal value, the roots being used as tonic. It is known for increasing the secretion and urination, used as mild laxative. The herb can be found growing in temperate regions of world and can be easily located in lawn, yards and roadsides. Dandelion grows in temperate region of Europe, Asia & North America. The plant has beautiful yellow flowers which looks really beautiful in gardens. The Dandelion herb help in curbing alcohol cravings due to withdrawal.[11] The roots of the Dandelion plant are used in curbing alcohol withdrawal related cravings. It is bitter in taste but it helps in increasing product of bile which in turn helps in treating alcoholism. The roots are crushed, boiled in water to extract the active ingradients, and filtered water extract is taken three times in a day to treat alcoholism.[11] Its roots stimulate appetite, leaves used as diuretics to help body to remove toxins from body. Thus it can be helpful in alcoholism treatment as it can protects liver and remove toxins from body. It also shows antioxidant source as it remove toxins from kidney, gall bladder and liver; and so improves immunity.

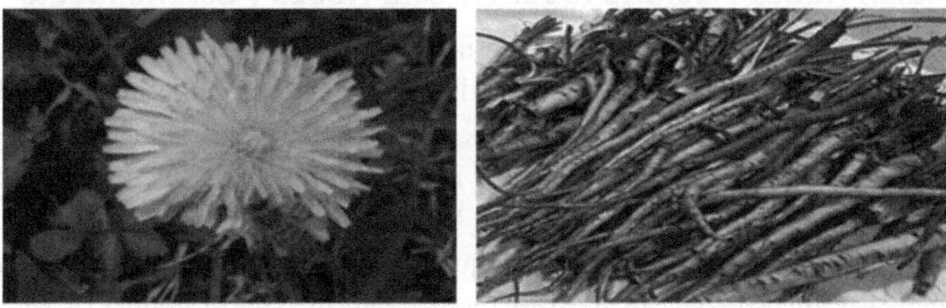

Fig. 2 Kanphool/Dandelion flower and roots (source: google images).

Brahmi – *Bacopa monnieri*

Brahmi is a Sanskrit word that refers to the feminine essence of universal consciousness as well as the creative potential that emerges from pure awareness. The Brahmi plant i.e. *Bacopa monnieri* is known in Ayurveda for its effect as brain tonic. Brahmi herb has a strong affinity for the lymph, blood, nervous tissue, and urinary tract, as well as the circulatory, digestive, and nervous systems. It is used in certain types of *vata* and *kapha* imbalances. Bacopa is suited for overall strengthening, energy promotion and said to support longevity. Brahmi is very supportive of the joints - clearing toxins while promoting comfort and freedom of movement. Mainly, Brahmi is known to rejuvenate the mind, enhance memory, improve concentration, to directly influence the quality of consciousness, and help to relax tension in the body.[12] As brain tonic and having effect on nervous system to bring to normal functioning, it help the alcoholic person in having better control on limb movements, body stamina and generating overall confidence in person towards the alcoholism treatment.

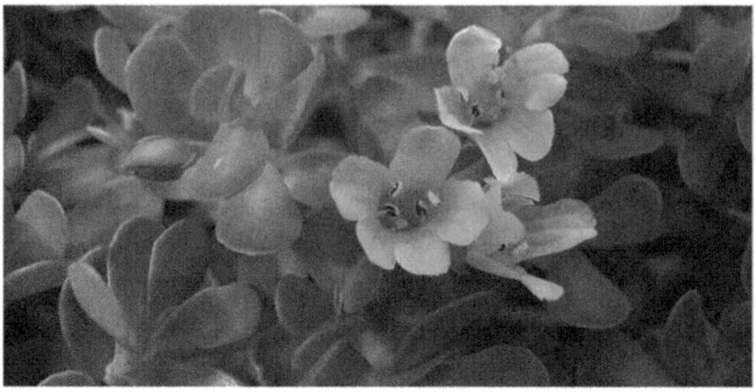

Fig. 3 Brahmi – *Bacopa monneiri* plant

Indian Kudzu *Pueraria tuberosa* and Kudzu *Pueraria lobata*

The Indian Kudzu known as Vidarikand in Sanskrit, the botanical name *Pueraria tuberosa* is a perenial woody climber and has tuberous roots. The plant bears white flowers with pink shade. Vidarikand is sweet in taste, heavy to digest, increases moisture level of tissues and have tremendous cooling properties. Medicinally, the Vidarikand is very useful in relieving constipation, boosts immunity, rejuvenates male reproductive system, increases quality (sperm motility) and quantity (sperm count) of semen, increases vitality. It is diuretic in nature, thus help in clearing toxins from body. It nourishes skin and rejuvenates the whole body.[13] Combined with many properties of Vidarikand like moisture increasing of tissues, diuretic and rejuvating properties, it is very effective in relieving alcohol craving.

The roots of Kudzu *Pueraria lobata* are also popular in China. It is a really popular herbal treatment that reduces alcohol cravings. People who are alcoholics should have kudzu roots in the form of kudzu drops in water or solid root power may be taken with warm water. Due to wide medicinal values, it may be taken daily and also as it does not have any harmful effects. The herb will fight alcoholism and over the time helps to get rid of alcohol cravings.

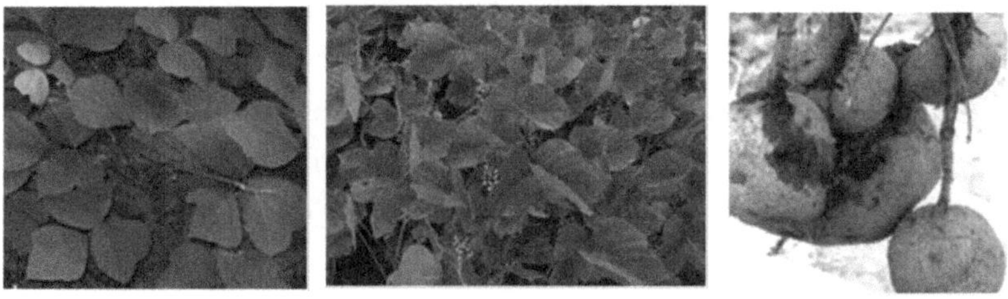

Fig. 4 Kudzu Plant, Indian Kudzu (Vidarikand) plant and roots

P. lobata Kudzu is helpful in lowering the hangover of alcohol. The hangover relieving impact is due to its diuretic and toxin removing properties. The kudzu suppresses intoxicating effects of alcohol after it entered the blood stream. Because of this, there is ancient claim that taking kudzu before drinking alcohol helped to stave off intoxication and hangovers.[14]

The medicinal value of Kudzu has been evaluated by modern scientific experimentations by researchers. Research evaluation of Kudzu extracts experimented on laboratory animals revealed that kudzu root extract help in the treatment of alcoholism.[14] The Kudzu is source of many isoflavonoids, such as daidzin and daidzein are the active isoflavonoids isolated from the kudzu. These isoflavanoids daidzin and daidzein have been reported by Keung and coworkers as alcohol preference suppressers in Syrian golden hamsters.[15] The anti-dipsotropic activity of daidzin have also been confirmed in different alcohol-drinking animal tests. Research studies results in different animals indicated that daidzin was effective in suppressing the craving for alcohol.

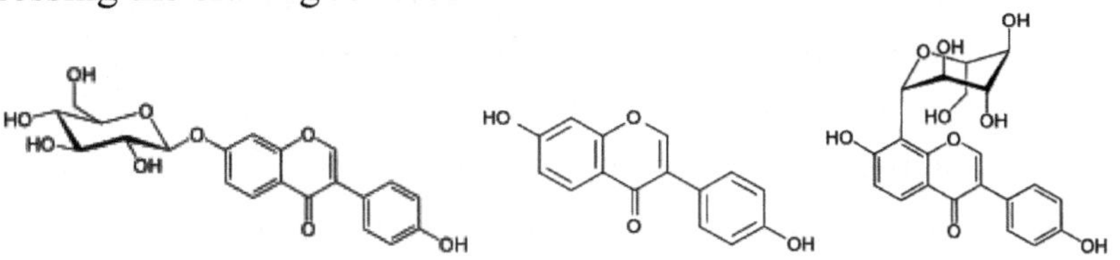

Fig. 5 Chemical structure of daidzin, daidzein and puerarin.

The puerarin, another isoflavanoid from Kudzu, have been reported to selectively reduce alcohol intake in alcohol-preferring rats. Puerarin is not as potent as daidzin. The puerarin showed reduced alcohol intake selectively after acute intraperitoneal administration.[16] Other investigations on the effects of *Radix Puerariae* and its major isoflavone puerarin on voluntary alcohol intake and alcohol withdrawal symptoms in P rats indicated that they suppressed alcohol drinking and withdrawal symptoms without entering the brain.[17] The absence of puerarin in plasma and the brain indicated the possibility that some non-specific mechanism might be involved in the anti-alcoholism effects of *Radix Puerariae* in P rats.

Keung & Vallee[18] found that compounds daidzin and prunetin seem to be particularly potent inhibitors of ALDH-2 in a comprehensive study involving examination of effect of a large number of flavonoids and isoflavonoids on the activities of both ALDH-1(mitochondria) and ALDH-2 (cytosol).[18] Further investigation of the inhibition reaction indicated that isoflavonoid prunetin was an allosteric inhibitor of ALDH-2. Though further studies are warranted towards evaluation of exact mechanism and target identification, the Kudzu roots powder or extract potentially help in reducing alcohol carving and treat alcoholism.

Ashwagandha – *withania somnifera*: *Withania somnifera,* commonly called Ashwagandha, is a small evergreen shrub of Solanaceae (Potato) family, attaining height upto 4-5 feet. It grow in dry regions of Asia (India, Srilanka, Pakistan), South Africa and Egypt. Ashwagaudha name comes from sanskrit word Ashave means horse, gandha- smell, as its roots smell like horse. It is popularly known as "Indian ginseng," because its biological effects are similar to those of Panax ginseng. In Ayurveda, *Withania somnifera* is a rasayana to treat physical-mental health, increase immunity, used as a tonic, aphrodisiac, sedative, and Medharasayana ('what promotes learning and a good memory') particularly for geriatric problems.[19] Withania somnifera has been widely used as a home remedy for a wide range of problems, including consumption, emaciation, debility, dyspepsia, and rheumatism, and its root is used to treat asthma.[20] This plant have alkaloids and steroids called as withanolides (withanferin A) which have strong anti-oxidant properties to slow down lipid peroxidant. Besides withaferin A, a large number of bioactive compounds can be obtained from *Withania somnifera*'s roots and leaves including 3-i-hydroxy-2, 3-dihydrowithanolideF, which show promising antibacterial and immunomodulating properties.

Withania somnifera is one important plants utilized in anti-addictive studies of drugs. The most common effect of *Withania somnifera* treatment is on withdrawal symptoms. Kulkarni and Ninan[21] reported that repeated administrations of *Withania somnifera* attenuated the development of tolerance to morphine's analgesic effects and suppressed morphine withdrawal jumps in animals.[21] *Withania somnifera* also attenuates several neurobiological changes induced by cold, hypoxia, or restraint stress in animals including the rise in plasma corticosterone levels, increases in dopaminergic receptor population in the corpus striatum, phagocytic index, and avdity index. The compounds sitoindosides VII-X, withaferin A showed increased superoxide dismutase catalysed glutathione peroxidise activity in front cortex of the brain 9 of rats) showing anti-stress effect. These anti-stress effects might reduce relapse in drug dependent patients. The precise mechanism for effects of *Withania somnifera* on morphine or other steroidal drug probably involves multiple neurotransmitters. For example, *Withania somnifera* blocks GABA binding to its receptors and increases chloride influx in the absence of GABA. It also down-regulates 5-HT1 and up-regulates 5-HT2 receptors, and inhibits calcium ion influx in glutaminergicion channels. Similar way *Withania somnifera* has potential for combating the withdrawal symptoms, cravings arsing due to treatment for alcoholism. Priya Bansal *et al* showed effect of Ashwagandha churna and shilajit on withdrawal symptoms of ethanol on rats.[22] Both withania plants (ashwagandha and shilajit) were found to be effective in dose dependent reduction of anxiety due to withdrawal symptoms after treating mice for 21 days with chronic consumption of alcohol, causing reduced GABA, serotonin level. As it acts as nerve tonic and improves functioning of central nervous system, it can be used in alone or in combination with other plant extracts for controlling or reducing withdrawal symptoms along with anti-addictive potential.[22,23]

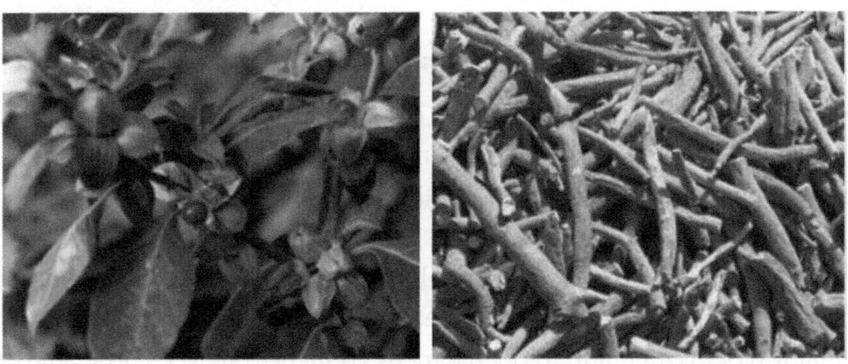

Fig. 6 Ashawagandha herb plant and roots

Herbs to treat sleep problems

The herbs that help in restoring the sleep also help in treatment of alcoholism as in ayurveda sleeplessness is considered to be one of the reason of alcohol consumption, and associated impact of alcoholism. Following herbs are recommended for sleep problems.

Jatamansi (*Nardostachys jatamansi*)

Jatamansi is a flowing plant with pink bell shaped flowers and found in Himalayans at an altitute of 3000-5000 meteres. The essential oil distilled from crushed Jatamansi rhizomes (underground stems) is used as perfume, and medicine to fight insomnia.[24]

Sarpgandha (*Rauvolfia serpentina*)

The sarpgandha or Indian snakeroot is a perennial flowing plant bearing beautiful red and white bud and flowers. The sarpgandha plant contains reserpine which was used as pharmaceutical drug to treat high blood pressure and disorders including schizophrenia. In controlled amount, the roots and leaves of sarpgandha are used for treating the lack of sleep (sleeplessness disorder).[25] It can be used to treat insomnia due to presence of indole alkaloid and it also show antihypertensive property. So it is helpful in relieving excited state of mind under the influence of alcohol.

Brahmi

As discussed above, Brahmi is used as tonic for brain and for the increasing the sleep in patients. It is considered as *sattvic* herbs relieving from mental aggravation. It has calming effect on nervous system enhances concentration, have effect on central nervous system.

Jaiphal/ Jaipatri (*Myristica fragrans*)

Jaiphal or Nutmeg is a spice used in cooking food. The powder of jaiphal is taken with milk or honey to improve the sleep, and curing sleeping disorders. It is used for improving the functioning of brain and treatment of Alzheimer disease. The jaiphal is also reported to release toxins from liver and kidneys. The excess of jaiphal may lead to nausea, hallucination and restlessness, so it should be taken on consultation with expert/doctor.[26] It is a natural detoxifier, anti toxic, balances *vaata* & cough. Its n-hexane extract is useful as antidepressant drug.

Herbs to Improve Liver Functions

The liver is the main organ affected due to heavy drinking. Fatty liver is mostly caused by large consumption of alcohol (it may also be caused by other factors, in which case it is termed as nonalcoholic fatty liver). The cells in the liver start retaining large amount of fat due to faulty abnormal metabolism within the liver. The liver supply fat to other organs as well as it removes the fat from blood released into it by other organs and tissues of the body. Restoring liver functioning to the normal is and should be an integral part of any alcoholism treatment. Many herbs have been mentioned in ayurveda texts that help in reversing the damage to liver caused by alcoholism, improve the functioning of liver, and help in bringing the liver to normal healthy state. The herbs Aloe Vera, Punarnava, Long pepper, Kutki and Tulsi are recommended for revival of liver health.[27]

Aloe Vera(*Aloe vera*) grows in tropical climates and is grown indoors as potted plants. The oral administration (aloe vera juice) is known to reduce blood glucose in diabetic patients and in lowering blood lipid level in hiperlipidaemia. The aloe vera help in digestion and keep the entire digestive tract detoxified and well functioning; thus assisting and supporting the functioning of liver. The anti-inflammatory nature of aloe vera relieve the inflammation of fatty liver cells and foster the functioning of liver.[28] Aloe vera boost immune system, it is also a natural source of vitamins B12.

Punarnava (*Boerhaavia diffusa*) with literal meaning 'bring back to life' or 'renewer' is creeper wild perenial herb found in India and Brazil. It grow throughout year except summer when it get dried. It bears small fleshy leaves, small white flower or reddish pink flowers, and fruits in winter. It is bitter in taste and has cooling effect. It has very high medicinal value. Punarnava is used for treatment of digestion, rejuvenates the body, and is diuretic. Punarnava is taken in liver problems, managing lipids and cholesterol in healthy limits and used in treatment of jaundice.[29]

Long pepper (*Piper longum*) commonly known as Pipli in India (Indian long pepper) is a flowering plant and its fruit, in dried form, is used as spice. It is known to increase digestion, and in ayurveda it is known to control vatta and kapha. It is used for treatment of enlarged liver (dried fruit is prescribed with honey) and also for jaundice.[30]

Kutki (Picrorrhiza kurroa) is found in Himalayan region and its root is used for the treatment of liver malfunctions. The ayurvedic texts have mentioned the use of Kutki as a good Pitta removing herb, Pacifies Pitta and Kapha conditions, and it has been recommended as very good liver tonic. The roots of Kutki is known for its Hepatoprotective properties, even in small doses it helps to cure various conditions like Lack of Appetite, Jaundice, and Bile disorders. It detoxifies the liver, blood and GI tract, and strengthens the liver. It helps to clear away the excessive fat deposits in liver, it helps in regulating and maintain the normal functions of the Liver. Kutki is also known for treatment of Cirrhosis of Liver.[31] It is known for its hepatoprotective properties. Kutki also reverse the hepatotoxic effect of drugs paracetamol and cure acute viral hepatitis.

Tulsi (*Ocimum sanctum*) is a popular herb commonly grown in home yards, pots in India. Its leaves are common additive to tea preparations. It is a good detoxifier and its daily consumption is said to prevent disease, promote general health, well being and longevity and assist in dealing with the stresses of daily life. Tulsi is also credited with giving luster to the complexion, sweetness to the voice and fostering beauty, intelligence, stamina and a calm emotional disposition.[32] The beneficial metabolic effects of tulsi are multiple and include protecting the liver, kidneys and pancreatic islet cells from free radical damage, enhancing liver bile acid synthesis and reducing liver lipid synthesis, and reducing inflammation.[33]

Amla (*phyllanthus emblica* family euphorbiaceae) juice is a very good source of carotene, iron and vitamin C. Also known as gooseberry, grown in atumn, its juice reduce obesity by increasing protein synthesis, reduce cholestrol thus reducing heart attack risk. Its juice also treat peptic ulcer, dysentery thus maintain liver fuctioning normal if taken with pure ghee twice daily. Amla is a natural blood purifier so it is natural detoxifier, increases haemoglobin, control blood sugar, anti-inflammatory, treat insomnia by taking with nutmeg powder. It is most easily available antioxidant source (superoxide dismutase). It strengthens lungs, liver, brain by removing free radicals, thus supports longevity.

Herbs to treat inflammation

Dashamoola: Dashamula is a traditional Ayurvedic formula for removing excess *Vata* from the body. The dashmoola is a mixture of roots of 10 medicinal plants: Bilva (*Aegle marmelos*), Agnimantha (*Premna mucronata*), Shyonaka (*Oroxylum indicum*), Patala (*Stereospermum suaveolens*), Gambhari (*Gmelina arborea*), Brihati (*Solanum indicum*), Kantakari (*Solanum xanthocarpum*), Gokshura (*Tribulus terrestris*), Shalaparni (*Desmodium gangeticum*), Prishnaparni (*Uraria picta*). The dashmoola is a nourishing muscle tonic that strengthens the body and calms the nerves. It has potent anti-inflammatory, antioxidant and moderate analgesic actions.[34] It is a part of several ayurvedic medicines and alone used for pain disorders and inflammatory diseases related to a musculoskeletal system including osteoarthritis, gouty arthritis, and rheumatoid arthritis.[34]

Herbal formula

E. Shanmugasundaram *et. al.* has developed pharmacological combination of 12 herbs by fermentation for treatment of alcoholism. The herbal formulation named as SKV was produced by fermentation of cane sugar with raisins and 12 Indian herbal ingredients. The formulation could bring down voluntary alcohol ingestion and increased food intake. It appeared to be a promising way to combat alcoholism.[35]

HOME REMEDIES

There are few home remedies that help the alcoholic person in ceasing alcohol consumption and combat withdrawal symptoms. It is concerned with the taking of selected foods in prescribed amount or pattern to tune up the biological cycle and demand leading to particular physiological action. Like there are some dietary components that have been reported to affect alcohol absorption from stomach or intestine. For example, vegetable oils such as soybean oil and coconut oil hold the alcohol that delay the elimination rate of gastric alcohol and thus reduces the chances of increase in plasma alcohol concentration. Soymilk products were reported to inhibit alcohol absorption in rats.[36] In addition, medicines from animals also contained many anti-alcohol substances such as pig and bovine bile. According to previous studies, bovine bile exerted its anti-intoxication effect by delaying gastric emptying time and inhibiting the absorption of alcohol in the intestinal tract. The taurine was identified to be the effective constituent in bovine bile responsible for anti-intoxication effect.[37]

Many other general food items help in reducing the impact of alcohol or help in reducing the desire for alcohol or lowers its impact (hangover etc). Few such remedial practices prescribed includes

1. Mix and powder the combination of coriander + capsicum + sugar flakes. Soak one teaspoon of this powder in a cup of water for eight hour. Filter it and take the filterate in the morning. It is a good *Antioxidant.*
2. A fresh lemon juice with sugar and pinch of salt (one lemon+sugar+pinch of salt mixed in one glass of water) when taken in the morning empty stomach, it act as good *Detoxifier.*
3. 20 grams of carom seeds should be boiled in 100 ml of water, filter, and take the filterate.
4. Taking any kind of sweet food item help to reduce the craving for alcohol.
5. The curd and yogurt are good Detoxifier and reduces the hangover.

6. One teaspoon of onion juice is recommended to reduce the hangover.
7. Consumption of juices reduces craving for alcohol. Take pomegranate or Apple or Grape juice at least two to three times a week. These contain antioxidants and slowly lower the desire for alcohol.
8. Include 10 gram of clarified butter (ghee) with sugar (*sakkar* – brown sugar) as food menu item. It is good general *antioxidant, and detoxifier, and reduces the craving for alcohol.*

NATUROPATHY TREATMENT

Naturopathy or naturopathic medicine is a form of pseudoscientific, alternative medicine that employs an array of practices branded as "natural", "non-invasive", and as promoting "self-healing." The ideology and methods of naturopathy are based on vitalism and self-healing.[38]

The naturopathy for alcoholism[39] involve reducing the food item, supplemented by juices (fruits and vegetable juices), and treatment with water and oil massages.[40] The dietry control is helpful in detoxification of body and slowly natural healing the craving for alcohol. The oil massage helps to strengthen nervous system, muscles, mental balance. It reduces stress. The Mud Bath strengthens, rejuvenates nervous system.[39]

Inclusion of Exercise (just warming up, avoiding much stress) and Yoga further improves memory, concentration, relieves tremors.[41]

General Routine Practices (Life style/Habit)

The person willing to leave alcohol drinking habit may adopt self practices which slowly can help in getting rid of alcoholism. These practices are self determined and practiced. Some of these practices do not have instant effect, however, over the time these might lead to a resolved impact.[42]

Simple general practices to get rid of alcoholism are:

- Take juice of pomegranate, grapes, watermelon and other water rich fruits.
- Avoid excess of non vegetarian food. Excess non veg food would increase *Rajas* and *Tamas* (as defined in Ayurveda), which may influence person to indulge in alcohol.
- Do not move out of home with empty stomach. Take your dinner (alcohol free) in early evening. When your stomach is full, you have less desire to have alcohol.

- Do not move out of home at night time. Staying at home help in getting engaged with family members.
- Do not join parties with alcoholic friends.
- Stay in contact with sober persons. Get engaged in general and social discussion (deviates the mind towards other activities).
- Take plenty of *sikanji* (water with sugar and little salt) at day time.
- Take sound and full length sleep. A sound sleep always rejuvinates your body. Being engaged in productive work help in good thinking and is one of sources for sound sleep.
- Think positively, avoid negative thinking. Think only for today, do not take tension for tomorrow (be stress free).
- Participate in social developmental activities.

STRESS DUE TO ALCOHOLISM (PSYCHOLOGICAL DISORDER)

Human brain contains a fluid called Dopamine. Alcoholism stimulates the brain to form (increase) synthesis of dopamine. The alcohol, thus, activates the nervous system and stimulates the precursors to promote dopamine formation, to keep and maintain dopamine level.

In the presence of alcohol, brain creates a receptor cells on its surface to learn the quantity and taste of alcohol. As the level of drinking increases, the receptor cells also increase in number. So when the person get less amount than desired (receptors), it start showing irritation; *i.e.* if there is insufficient level of alcohol, the receptor cells become aggressive and agitating to have the regular level of alcohol, and entice the person for sufficient alcohol level. After treatment, when a person stops drinking, again all cells but only few become receptive to get same doses. If they are not fulfilled by regular quantity, they creates huge craving.

Treatment of alcoholism allopathy is always accompanied by many side effects like increasing heartbeat, palpitations, nausea, vomiting, headache as well as sedation. Use of herbal medicine can be potent therapeutic measure to control above problem. The herbs such as ashawgandha, kanphool etc and their formulations discussed above help in combating the withdrawal stress.

ALCOHOL METABOLISM AND DETOXIFICATION

Alcohol metabolism is concerned with conversion of ethyl alcohol present in blood stream to other products through biochemical pathways in particular organs of body. The detoxification is removal or lowering of amount of ethyl alcohol or its metabolites from blood through direct excretion or conversion into other products. Ethyl alcohol is removed from the body mainly by metabolism in the liver. Approximately 90% of the alcohol is metabolized in the liver by alcohol dehydrogenase (ADH) followed by aldehyde dehydrogenase (ALDH), while the gastrointestinal tract, lungs and kidneys play only a minor role. Liver is main organ that is damaged due to heavy drinking over the time. Because alcohol-metabolizing enzymes such as ADH, ALDH and the microsomal alcohol oxidizing system (MEOS) contributed to the clearance of alcohol and toxic acetaldehyde, the synthetic chemical drugs or herbs substances that stimulated these enzyme activities were expected to ameliorate alcohol toxicity. The most of radical developments or research efforts for development of alcohol deaddiction or hangover combating formulations oriented towards the development of alcohol-metabolizing enzymes stimulant. Targeting the enhanced activity of ADH, ALDH or MEOS was one of the strategies for developing an alcoholism remedy or hangover lowering. Some attempts were made to develop an effective alcohol metabolic stimulant from natural dietary components and herbs. Many of the food constituents and herbal extracts are found to be active stimulants of these enzymes. For example, sesamin, garlic and soymilk products[36] were found to be effective natural hangover remedies, which enhance alcohol metabolism and acetaldehyde clearance. Many herbs formulations have detoxifying properties and thus find application in alcoholism treatment.

The Kidney is not a alcohol metabolism organ, however, it help in lowering the amount of alcohol from blood through excretion. The herbs that have diuretic properties also help in detoxifying the alcohol by direct excretion. The Kudzu roots (discussed above) have such effect.

OTHER GLOBAL HERBAL DRUGS

Besides above discussed herb formulations, there a number of herbs that has been used in traditional medicines for alcoholism treatment in different countries. The prominent selected herbs used for hangover, detoxification and alcohol carving have been included below.

Ginseng *Panax ginseng*

Ginseng is a popular herbal remedy for treating alcoholism, particularly in China and Korea. It has several beneficial properties which **helps in energizing and revitalizing**. It helps in detoxification of alcohol from the body which in turn helps in treatment of alcoholism. It is used by alcoholics to get rid of alcohol cravings. The ginseng roots are boiled in water and filtered, and then this ginseng roots water extract is taken daily for alcoholism treatment. The effects of Panax ginseng on blood alcohol clearance have been assessed by orally administering alcohol (3.2 g/kg) and aqueous extract of red ginseng to rats. The presence of ginseng significantly lowered the concentration of alcohol in the blood; however, contrary to that intraperitoneal injection of ginseng extract had no effect on level of alcohol in blood. These results indicated that ginseng exerted its anti-intoxication effect by inhibiting GastroIntestinal tract absorption of alcohol.43

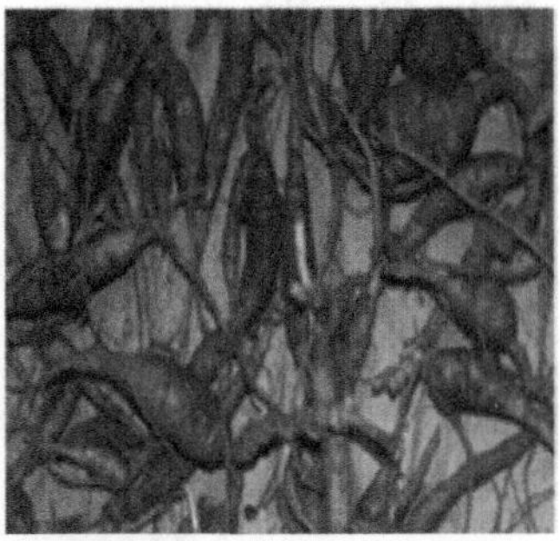

Fig. 7 Roots of Ginseng Panax ginseng. Source: google images.

Heavy drinking results in hangover symptoms as action of alcohol dehydrogenase converts into acetaldehyde then it is metabolized into acetate due to enzymatic action of dehydrogenase enzyme. This plant helps in easing alcohol metabolism.

Opuntia plant *opuntia fragilis* or *ficus indica* (belonging to cactaceae family), also known as prickly pear with spines, is useful in treating inflammation problem due to drinking.

Passion Flower

Passion flower is used as a herbal treatment for withdrawing alcohol completely. Passion flower help to stop craving for alcohol. It is used in homeopathic medicine to treat insomnia & stress related problems, and anxiety. Alcohol ingestion results in all above problems if person think of quitting, in

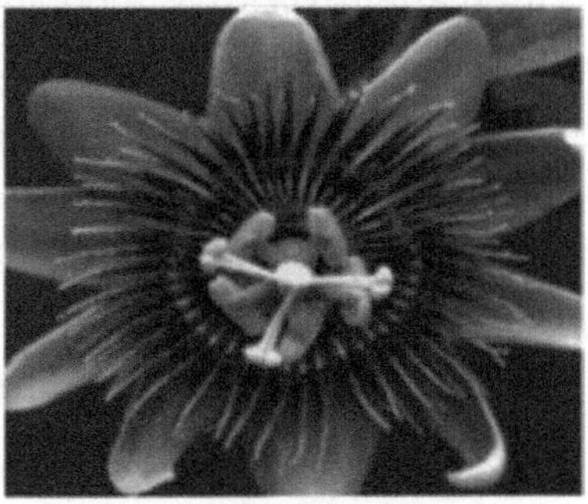

Fig. 8 Passion Flower.

form of withdrawal symptoms. Clinical trial on mice of this flower extrtact reduced withdrawal anxiety to 90% as compared to no treatment control.

Milk Thistle

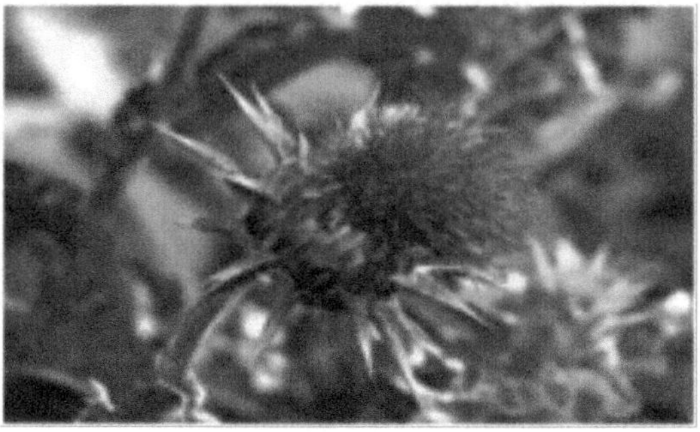

Fig. 9 Milk Thistle plant.

Milk Thistle is an effective herbal remedy which cures many health conditions such as gall bladder and liver disorders. **Excess of alcohol can cause damage to liver** and milk thistle is a herb which cures liver conditions.

For lowering the hangover, a number of herbs such as *Radix Puerariae*, *FlosPuerariae* and *Hovenia dulcis* are used. In addition, many other natural products such as ginseng, mung bean, ricebean, radish and dandelion are used as hangover remedies in folk medicine. In Korea, the herb Virgate Wormwood is known to be tremendously effective in expelling accumulated alcohol from the body. It removes toxic wastes from the blood and organs and promotes urination. Because of this, doctors of oriental medicine prescribe the herb widely for liver diseases. In Mexico, a common hangover remedy consists of alfalfa seed and dried orange tree leaves, steeped in one cup of boiled water. In Brazil, the herb jurubeba (*Solanum paniculatum*) is the most popular hangover remedy, which is used after excessive food and alcohol consumption to alleviate indigestion and bloating in the stomach. It has been proved that this herb is helpful in the treatment of liver diseases such as chronic hepatitis, liver obstruction and swelling of the liver. In Egypt, cabbage with vinegar is considered as an effective hangover remedy. It is believed that cabbage consumption allows drinkers to drink more alcoholic beverages.

St John's wort *Hypericum perforatum, hypericaceae family*

The extracts of H. perforatum (St John's wort) have been shown to reduce voluntary intake of alcohol significantly.[44,45] This herb have anti depressant and antiinflammatory property as an arachidonate 5-lipoxygenase inhibitor and cox-1 inhibitor. It is a good anti depressant with minimum side-effects. Its major constituents hyperforin shows anti-inflammatory and neurotrophic activity.

Tabernathe Iboga (family *apocynaceae*)

The root bark of the African shrub *Tabernathe iboga* has an indole alkaloids Ibogaine, which was found to significantly reduce volitional alcohol consumption in alcohol-preferring rats. Ibogaine exerted its anti-craving effects on voluntary alcohol intake by interacting with the brain systems involved instimulating dopaminergic and serotonergic systems.46 Ibogaine is naturally occuring psychoactive substance found in this plant. It is commonly used in addiction problem in Africa. It is cardiotoxic, so not approved as drug as it leads to ataxia, nausea, vomiting, degeneration of cardiac muscles.

A number of herb or their extracts has been shown to reduce the gastrointestinal absorption of alcohol in experimental settings. These include *Panax notoginseng*(Burk.), *Acanthopanax gracilistylus*, *Panaxquinquefolium* L., *Aralia elata* [63], *Sapindusmukurossi* (Japanese soapnut tree), the seeds of *Aesculus hippocastanum* (horse chestnuttree) and *Camellia japonica*, fruit of *Kochia scoparia*, leaves of *Laurusnobilis* (bay leaf).

Hovenia dulcis herb is known to be effective in alleviating lingering intoxication. *H. dulcis* is reported to decrease alcohol concentration remarkably in blood and promote the clearance of alcohol.[47]

SUMMARY

In summary, the different herbs formulations have potential to treat the alcoholism and associated diseases. We can use plant parts—their extracts, juices etc. to cure addiction related problems potentially. The treatment of alcoholism is accompanied by withdrawal symptoms along with many worse effect of alcohol consumption on liver, nervous system, cognitive ability, limb movement & associated socialistic behavioural changes in addicted person. So taking into account of all above health problems, herbal treatment to detoxify, improving mental health, and to treat this alarming problem is highly useful. Herbal treatment combined with alternative medicines is useful in combating psychological problem, detoxification of addicted person to minimize withdrawal craving symptoms, and thus helpful in getting rid of addiction and leads to increased longevity.

REFERENCES

1. C. Cui, A. Noronha, H. Morikawa, V.A. Alvarez, G.D. Stuber, K.K. Szumlinski, T.L. Kash, M. Roberto, M.V. Wilcox. New insights on neurobiological mechanisms underlying alcohol addiction. *Neuropharmacology* **2013**, 67, 223-32.
2. C.B.D. Soto, W.E. O'Donnell, L.J. Allred, C.E. Lopes. Symptomatology in alcoholics at various stages of abstinence. *Alcoholism: Clinical and Experimental Research* **1985**, 9, 505-12.
3. W.H. Organization. Cough and cold remedies for the treatment of acute respiratory infections in young children. **2001**.
4. S. Sekar, S. Mariappan. Traditionally fermented biomedicines, arishtas and asavas from Ayurveda. **2008**.
5. R. Verma. Alcoholism in Ayurveda. *Quarterly journal of studies on alcohol* **1950**, 11, 484.
6. S.K. Shetty, H. Savitha. Critical Review on role of Panchakarma in Madatyaya (Alcoholic Disorders). *Journal of Ayurveda and Holistic Medicine (JAHM)* **2013**, 1, 12-16.
7. T.L. Devaraj. The panchakarma treatment of Ayurveda, Dhavantari Oriental Publications, **1980**.
8. G.S. Acharya. Panchakarma illustrated, Chaukhamba Sanskrit Pratishthan Delhi, **2006**; Vol. 72.
9. A.K. Sharma Panchakarma therapy in ayurvedic medicine. In Scientific Basis for Ayurvedic Therapies; CRC Press: **2003**, pp 43-61.
10. M. Heba, S. Faraz, S. Banerjee. Effect of shankhpushpi on alcohol addiction in mice. *Pharmacognosy Magazine* **2017**, 13, S148.
11. Y. You, S. Yoo, H.-G. Yoon, J. Park, Y.-H. Lee, S. Kim, K.-T. Oh, J. Lee*et. al.* In vitro and in vivo hepatoprotective effects of the aqueous extract from Taraxacum officinale (dandelion) root against alcohol-induced oxidative stress. *Food and chemical toxicology* **2010**, 48, 1632-37.
12. H. Singh, B. Dhawan. Neuropsychopharmacological effects of the Ayurvedic nootropic Bacopa monniera Linn.(Brahmi). *Indian journal of Pharmacology* **1997**, 29, 359.
13. N.V. Rao, B. Pujar, S. Nimbal, S. Shantakumar, S. Satyanarayana. Nootropic activity of tuber extract of Pueraria tuberosa (Roxb). **2008**.
14. N.R. McGregor. Pueraria lobata (Kudzu root) hangover remedies and acetaldehyde-associated neoplasm risk. *Alcohol* **2007**, 41, 469-78.
15. G.-Y. Gao, D.-J. Li, W.M. Keung. Synthesis of daidzin analogues as potential agents for alcohol abuse. *Bioorganic & medicinal chemistry* **2003**, 11, 4069-81.

16. D.M. Penetar, C.J. Teter, Z. Ma, M. Tracy, D.Y.-W. Lee, S.E. Lukas. Pharmacokinetic profile of the isoflavone puerarin after acute and repeated administration of a novel kudzu extract to human volunteers. *Journal of Alternative & Complementary Medicine* **2006**, 12, 543-48.

17. E. Benlhabib, J.I. Baker, D.E. Keyler, A.K. Singh. Effects of purified puerarin on voluntary alcohol intake and alcohol withdrawal symptoms in P rats receiving free access to water and alcohol. *Journal of medicinal food* **2004**, 7, 180-86.

18. W.-M. Keung, B.L. Vallee. Daidzin: a potent, selective inhibitor of human mitochondrial aldehyde dehydrogenase. *Proceedings of the National Academy of Sciences* **1993**, 90, 1247-51.

19. A. Nandkarni. Indian Materia Medica Popular Prakashan Bombay Vol I&II (reprinted). **1982**.

20. R. Archana, A. Namasivayam. Antistressor effect of Withania somnifera. *Journal of ethnopharmacology* **1998**, 64, 91-93.

21. S.K. Kulkarni, I. Ninan. Inhibition of morphine tolerance and dependence by Withania somnifera in mice. *Journal of ethnopharmacology* **1997**, 57, 213-17.

22. P. Bansal, S. Banerjee. Effect of withinia somnifera and shilajit on alcohol addiction in mice. *Pharmacognosy Magazine* **2016**, 12, S121.

23. M. Prabhu, A. Rao, K. Karanth. Neuropharmacological activity of Withania somnifera. *Fitoterapia* **1990**, 61, 237-40.

24. A. Singh, A. Kumar, S. Duggal. Nardostachys jatamansi DC. potential herb with CNS effects. *Asian Journal of Pharmaceutical Research and Health Care* **2009**, 1, 276-90.

25. R. Badhwar, G. Karira, S. Ramaswami. Rauwolfia serpentina-the Wonder Drug of India (Rauwolfia, Sarpagandha). *Indian Forester* **1955**, 81, 258-68.

26. C. Van Gils, P.A. Cox. Ethnobotany of nutmeg in the Spice Islands. *Journal of ethnopharmacology* **1994**, 42, 117-24.

27. A. Subramoniam, P. Pushpangadan. Development of phytomedicines for liver disease. *Indian journal of Pharmacology* **1999**, 31, 166.

28. Y. Cui, Q. Ye, H. Wang, Y. Li, W. Yao, H. Qian. Hepatoprotective potential of Aloe vera polysaccharides against chronic alcohol□induced hepatotoxicity in mice. *Journal of the Science of Food and Agriculture* **2014**, 94, 1764-71.

29. D. Bhowmik, K.S. Kumar, S. Srivastava, S. Paswan, A.S. Dutta. Traditional Indian Herbs Punarnava and Its Medicinal Importance. *Journal of Pharmacognosy and Phytochemistry* **2012**, 1, 52-57.

30. S. Jalalpure, M. Patil, N. Prakash, K. Hemalata, F. Manvi. Hepatoprotective activity of the fruits of piper longum linn. *Indian journal of pharmaceutical sciences* **2003**, 65, 363.
31. A. Vaidya, D. Antarkar, J. Doshi, A. Bhatt, V. Ramesh, P. Vora, D. Perissond, A. Baxi, P. Kale. Picrorhiza kurroa (Kutaki) Royle ex Benth as a hepatoprotective agent-experimental & clinical studies. *Journal of postgraduate medicine* **1996**, 42, 105.
32. M.M. Cohen. Tulsi - Ocimum sanctum: A herb for all reasons. *Journal of Ayurveda and Integrative Medicine* **2014**, 5, 251-59.
33. T. Suanarunsawat, W.D. Ayutthaya, T. Songsak, S. Thirawarapan, S. Poungshompoo. Lipid-lowering and antioxidative activities of aqueous extracts of Ocimum sanctum L. leaves in rats fed with a high-cholesterol diet. *Oxid Med Cell Longev* **2011**, 962025, 21.
34. R.R. Parekar, S.S. Bolegave, P.A. Marathe, N.N. Rege. Experimental evaluation of analgesic, anti-inflammatory and anti-platelet potential of Dashamoola. *Journal of Ayurveda and Integrative Medicine* **2015**, 6, 11.
35. E. Shanmugasundaram, K.R. Shanmugasundaram. An Indian herbal formula (SKV) for controlling voluntary ethanol intake in rats with chronic alcoholism. *Journal of ethnopharmacology* **1986**, 17, 171-82.
36. M. Kano, F. Ishikawa, S. Matsubara, H. Kikuchi-Hayakawa, Y. Shimakawa. Soymilk products affect ethanol absorption and metabolism in rats during acute and chronic ethanol intake. *The Journal of nutrition* **2002**, 132, 238-44.
37. K. Taxhiyshiki, K. Imaizumi. Lowering and delaying actions of bovine bile on plasma ethanol levels in rats. *Journal of nutritional science and vitaminology* **1992**, 38, 69-82.
38. S.A. Fleming, N.C. Gutknecht. Naturopathy and the primary care practice. *Primary Care: Clinics in Office Practice* **2010**, 37, 119-36.
39. J.E. Barker. Natural medicine approaches in the treatment of alcoholism. *Townsend Letter: The Examiner of Alternative Medicine* **2007**, 124-28.
40. H. Rajput. Treatment of Chronic Alcoholism: An Integrated Approach. *Alternative & Integrative Medicine* **2014**, 1-4.
41. S. Chougala, P. Shetty, H. Shashikiran, C. Kumar, S. Biswagar. A Study on Influence of Yoga on Balance and Gait Deficits among Alcoholics. *International Journal of Innovative Research and Development|| ISSN 2278–0211* **2015**, 4.
42. K. Dean. Self-care components of lifestyles: the importance of gender, attitudes and the social situation. *Social Science & Medicine* **1989**, 29, 137-52.

43. M. Yeo, D.-K. Kim, S.W. Cho, H. Do Hong. Ginseng, the root of Panax ginseng CA Meyer, protects ethanol-induced gastric damages in rat through the induction of cytoprotective heat-shock protein 27. *Digestive diseases and sciences* **2008**, 53, 606-13.

44. I. Panocka, M. Perfumi, S. Angeletti, R. Ciccocioppo, M. Massi. Effects of Hypericum perforatum extract on ethanol intake, and on behavioral despair: a search for the neurochemical systems involved. *Pharmacology Biochemistry and Behavior* **2000**, 66, 105-11.

45. A.H. Rezvani, D. Overstreet, Y. Yang, E. Clark. Attenuation of alcohol intake by extract of Hypericum perforatum (St John's wort) in two different strains of alcohol-preferring rats. *Alcohol and Alcoholism* **1999**, 34, 699-705.

46. J.R. Donnelly. The need for ibogaine in drug and alcohol addiction treatment. *The Journal of legal medicine* **2011**, 32, 93-114.

47. B.-J. Xu, Y.-Q. Deng, X.-Q. Jia, J.-H. Lee, E.-K. Mo, H.-J. Kang, C.-K. Sung. A rapid screening for alcohol detoxification constituents of Hovenia dulcis by microplate reader. *Journal of Applied Biological Chemistry* **2003**, 46, 105-09.

Editors' Note

The de-addiction therapies have different mode of operation. The chemical drugs might have side effect on patients, so the alternative medicines play a major role in de-addiction of an alcoholic without inducing side effects. The alternative medicine, mainly the herbal based Ayurvedic medicines, are highly useful as alcohol de-addiction therapy. The different herbal drugs formulation and combinations have varied impact on the body, so an alternative therapy should be followed in guidance of experts in field.

❑❑❑

8

Psychopharmacotherapy for Alcoholism: Challenges in Novel Approaches

Rahmat Bano* and Ravinder Singh**

Abstract

Alcoholism is a chronic relapsing disorder which develops the risk of physical, psychological, socioeconomic and legal problems. From the literature many pharmacotherapeutic approaches are being experimented on alcohol dependents for their efficacy and safety till date in preclinical and clinical setups. Significant pharmacotherapeutic improvement in percentage of success are achieved in terms of maintaining frequency and quantity of consumption when combination therapeutic regime of psychopharmacotherapies is adopted which reflects positive results in psychosocial behaviour along with anticraving relapse maintenance. Therefore, Pharmacotherapy could be more effective in multimodal approach including psychological and social support. This chapter is a narration about many brain neurotransmitter systems (CNS) activities with various phases of addiction currently being used for pharmacotherapies and psychopharmacotherapies along with co-morbid disorders for treatment of alcoholism. Several FDA approved drugs and drugs with conjunct therapy and combination therapy are discussed.

*Division of Innovations and Transnational Research (ITR), ICMR, New Delhi. India
**DIVISION OF NON COMMUNICABLE DISEASES (NCD) , ICMR, New Delhi. India

However, there is still a need to decipher the most effective therapeutic approaches concomitantly to deal with alcohol dependency. Alcohol withdrawal syndrome is also a challenge to deal for willing outpatient and inpatient for primary healthcare physicians to maintain the abstinence, execute detoxification and achieve relapse. To address more effective therapeutic approach various new combination of pharmacotherapeutic and psychopharmacotherapeutic therapies along with psychiatric co-morbid approaches are being in experimentation in preclinical and clinical research as registered on primary registries worldwide.

Keywords: Alcohol dependency, Pharmacotherapy, Psychopharmacotherapy, Psychiatric Co-morbidity, Novel Approaches

INTRODUCTION

Alcohol addiction is alarming revelation, which is drastically increasing few folds every year, which is increasing social, spiritual, mental, emotional and legal problems by adding alcohol users including male, females, adolescents, students and other users. Holistic approach to treat alcoholism is the need-of-hour, as over 38% of global population above 15 years consumes alcohol. Every year the per capita consumption of alcohol is rebounding which leads to socioeconomic burden and health consequences of alcohol addicted population. As a result liver cirrhosis, acetic, stroke, behavioural misbalance, cancer patients are increasing significantly every year. Undoubtedly, increase in the number of road accidents, casualties, injuries, assault, violence, suicide, murders etc. are evident in media. Other mental health concerns like personality disorders, depression, anxiety and seizures are mounting every year. Prevalence of underage drinking alcohol is again a cause of concern which is more common in children of alcoholic parents, which affects the adolescent brain development and increase the risk of binge drinking and Alcohol Use Disorders (AUD). Also drastically, the number of female consumers of alcohol have increased, which leads to family consequences, miscarriages, Fatal Alcohol Syndrome (FAS) and neurological disorders in developing child in pregnant females. Number of college students, aged 18-22 years consuming alcohol, are escalating remarkably day-by-day, which is leading to unintentional injuries viz. motor vehicle crashes, assaulting other students, sexual abuse. Also, includes, missing classes, lowering the grades and falling in classes which disturbs the class.

Globally, more than two billion people consume alcohol and around 76 million are diagnosed as alcohol dependent. More than 60 types of medical health problems, casualties and injuries are being known to be associated by alcohol dependency.[1] The prevalence of alcohol use and abuse varies across the countries depending upon their socio-cultural milieu and practise. In India, epidemiological markers such as hospitalization, death due to cirrhosis and sales of alcohol clearly indicates blueprint of enhancing consumption of alcohol. However, patterns of drinking and types of medical health conditions due to alcoholism differ markedly throughout the globe.[2]

Definition

Alcohol addiction is a chronic relapsing condition with a multifactorial variability in drinking prototype which has no marked difference between social or occasional drinker chronic or dangerous drinker. Alcohol Dependence Syndrome is a psychiatric condition and physiological problem. The very first definition of alcohol dependency was published by Griffith Edwards and Milton Gross in 1976, which describe the provisionally outlined and argued for a new conceptual understanding of alcohol dependence, which is based upon the idea of dependence as a syndrome.[3] The principals of ADS were hastily adopted by World Health Organisation (WHO) and classified the basics of alcohol and drugs problems in the International Classification of Diseases (ICD-10) and the Diagnostic and Statistical Manual (DSM-IV) of the American Psychiatric Association. Hence, the diagnostic guidelines of WHO in 1992 of ADS derived were in three or more criterion showed for dependency out of these given criteria are: (i) Strong desire for alcohol or substance; (ii) Problem in defining the limits like onset or level of consumptions; (iii) Limiting the use of alcohol or reduces the consumption which states physiological withdrawal; (iv) Tolerance of alcohol effects which increases intake to reach the effect levels of the lower intake; (v) When the recovery from the effects of alcohol prolongs; and (vi) Damaging results due to over consumption and the user is aware about it. However, ICD-10 has come up with the concept of "Harmful Use" to describe who do not fulfil the definition of dependence syndrome and still have problems because of consumption of alcohol.[4]

Signs and Symptoms of Alcohol Abuse

Severe medical symptoms due to progressive alcohol consumption leads to negative consequences including alcohol abuse are: (i) No control on drinking once started; (ii) Becoming irresponsible towards family and profession; (iii) Harmful behaviour which result in legal, financial and/or health consequences for themselves and others; (iv) In unfavourable condition uncontrolled anger and/or other harmful emotions; and (v) Insomnia could be due to oversleeping.

Signs and Symptoms of Alcohol Dependence

Alcohol dependency is inability to quit drinking alcohol and body becomes physically addicted and mentally dependent which reflects following symptoms: (i) Considerable hangovers to recover from after effects of alcohol use; (ii) Increased tolerance due to higher consumption of alcohol; (iii) Irresponsible towards family and profession; (iv) Acknowledgement of side effects of medication given to reduce effects of alcohol consumption; and (v) Withdrawal symptoms when unable to consume alcohol. Nevertheless, uncontrolled drinking of alcohol is characterised by physical dependency and inability to discontinue regardless knowing about serious consequences.

CURRENT PHARMACOTHERAPIES

The current Pharmacotherapies focus primarily on reduction on alcohol use (anticraving agents), overdose prevention, alcohol withdrawal management, detoxification, relapse prevention and maintenance. Psychopharmacotherapies, adjunct therapies and treatment with co-morbid condition along with alcohol dependency are also in focus these days. For all the therapeutic approaches for the patient of alcohol dependency in outpatient and inpatient hospital setup a personalized approach towards patient is needed and specialized trained clinicians would be more effective in the treatment of such population. Few terms are commonly used and need to be understood like: Alcohol withdrawal (AW) symptoms, Alcohol Withdrawal Syndrome (AWS) and Detoxification which are explained later in this chapter.

The compilation of current Pharmacotherapies, Psychopharmacotherapies and Psychiatric Co-morbid Disorders are narrated in Table 1 for quick reference. All the drugs in Table 1 are already been approved by FDA.

These drugs are been used in inpatient and outpatient setup to treat alcohol dependence, Psychiatric Co-morbidity with alcoholism and/or for other symptomatic and physiological disorders associated with alcoholism. All the subheads are explained separately for better understanding.

Table 1: Current Pharmacotherapies, Psychopharmacotherapies for Alcohol Dependency & Psychiatric Comorbidity

Medication	Dosage	Mechanism of action and target receptors	Pathways	Drug indication	*References
Naltrexone	Tablets 25 mg, 50 mg and 100 mg/day Extended – release injectable suspension : 380 mg/vial	μ, κ and δ competitive antagonist	opioid	Prescribed Drug – FDA approved drug: Reduces cravings and diminishes the effects of alcohol and Opioids. Extended – release injectable indicate for prevention of relapse to Opioids or alcohol.	5 & 6
Methadone	Tablet: 5 mg, 10 mg Tablet for suspension: 40 mg Oral concentrate: 10 mg/mL, Oral solution: 5 mg/5 ml, 10 mg/5mL Injection :10 mg/mL	μ, agonist and also possible antagonist at N-methyl-D-Asparate receptor		Prescribed drug – FDA approved drug : Reduces craving for Opioid dependency. Alcohol dependency is studied scantily.	6 & 7
Nalmefene	Tablet: 10 mg and 40 mg / day; 20 or 80 mg / day to heavy drinking	μ, κ and δ competitive antagonist		Prescribed drug: FDA approved drug. Has anticraving effects, Longer half-life, greater oral bioavailability, and no observed dose-dependent liver toxicity compared to Naltrexone.	5, 8, & 9

Contd...

Medication	Dosage	Mechanism of action and target receptors	Pathways	Drug indication	*References
Haloperidol	Used in combination therapy (Not approved by FDA for geriatric patients)	D2-antagonist	dopamine	Prescribed drug: FDA approved drug. Anti-psychotic pre-treatment with haloperidol significantly reduced alcohol craving, amount of alcohol ingested, and reduced impulsivity. In alcohol abuse rapid sedation should be initiated with a high-potency anti-psychotic drug such as Haloperidol (Haldol) at 5-10 mg PO or IM, frequently given with anticholinergics, Benztropine (Cogentin) (1-2 mg) or Diphenhydramine (Benadryl) (25-50 mg); both can be given PO or IM to prevent extrapyramidal adverse effects.	5, 10 & 11
Aripiprazole	Dosage as per Adjunct therapy and combination therapy	D2 and 5-HT1A/2C partial agonist 5-HT2A antagonist	dopamine	Prescribed Drug: antipsychotic, reduce craving, but to a lesser extent than with Naltrexone. FDA approved for the treatment of schizophrenia and acute manic and mixed episodes of bipolar disorder and as an adjunct for the treatment of major depressive disorder.	5 & 12

Contd...

Medication	Dosage	Mechanism of action and target receptors	Pathways	Drug indication	*References
Quetiapine	Dosage as per Adjunct therapy and combination therapy	D1-2 antagonist 5-HT1A partial agonist 5-HT2A antagonist adrenergic α1-2 antagonist		Prescribed Drug: FDA approved drug. Improves abstinence, reduces craving, and psychiatric symptom intensity. Drug used in bipolar disorder and therapy for heavy drinker.	5 & 13
Olanzapine	Dosage as per Adjunct therapy and combination therapy (2.5 and 5 mg are studied	D2,4 and 5-HT2 antagonist		FDA approved drug: pharmacogenomic approach targets the effect of craving in heavy drinking alcoholics.	5 & 14
Ondansetron	Dosage as per Adjunct therapy and combination therapy	5-HT3 antagonist	serotonin	Prescribed drug: FDA approved drug. Beneficial effects in reducing drinking behaviour in early onset drinkers; Naltrexone and Ondansetron, alone or in combination, decreased alcohol cue-induced activation.	5
Fluoxetine	20 mg/day for the first two weeks then 40 mg/day if necessary	serotonin-specific reuptake inhibitor (SSRI)		Not potential drug: Reduces craving but not for long.	5 & 15
Buspirone	10- 20 mg divided into two/three daily doses, was shown to be useful in alcohol-detoxification.	serotonin agonist		Prescribed drug: FDA approved drug for anxiety, relax skeletal muscles, induce sleep and detoxification.	16

Contd...

Medication	Dosage	Mechanism of action and target receptors	Pathways	Drug indication	*References
Topiramate	Tablets : initial 25 mg/day; maintenance 300 mg/day in divided doses	α-amino-3-hydroxy-5-methyl-4-isoxazolepropionic acid receptor (AMPA)/kainate glutamate antagonist gamma-amino butyric acid (GABA) a agonist carbonic anhydrase enzyme antagonist	inhibition	FDA approved drug. Used for alcoholics as Adjunct therapy: antiepileptic drug and anticonvulsants, decreased craving but not much, improved quality of life, however, genotypic side effects Prescribed drug : FDA approved drug. Reduces craving, anti-epileptic medications, adjunct therapy, In combination with Clozapine, lamotrigine was shown to reduce craving among patients suffering from schizophrenia and co-morbid alcohol dependence FDA approved drug for partial onset of seizers. and adjunct therapy for detoxification of alcohol. Newer antiepileptic agent Drug indication : FDA approved drug for seizers Zonisamide is safe and well tolerated in this sample and associated with improvement in alcohol craving and alcohol consumption in adjunct therapy. Prescribed drug: FDA approved drug for relief of flexor spasms, concomitant pain and muscular rigidity. Easy to manage, and rare euphoria, craving and other pleasant effects (Studies are undergoing)	5, 17 & 18

Contd...

Medication	Dosage	Mechanism of action and target receptors	Pathways	Drug indication	*References
Lamotrigine	Tablet : 5 and 15mg/kg	sodium channel blocker		Reduce alcohol craving. GHB is a naturally occurring substance that is approved for restricted use by the FDA to treat narcolepsy. GHB has also been used as a general anesthetic and to treat conditions such as insomnia, clinical depression and alcoholism	5 & 19
Levetiracetam	Used as per adjunct therapy Undergoing Trials are registered https://clinicaltrials.gov/ct2/show/NCT00325182	not fully elucidated, but it has been found to target high-voltage, N-type calcium channels, the synaptic vesicle protein 2A (SV2A)			5 & 20
Zonisamide	50 mg/d and titrated to a maximum dose of 300 mg/d	modulation of voltage-gated ion channels, enhancement of synaptic inhibition, and inhibition of synaptic excitation			5 & 21
Baclofen	15 mg/day for the first three days and 30 mg/day for the subsequent four weeks, (used in combination therapy)	GABA agonist			5, 15, 22 & 23
Gamma-hydroxy-butyric acid (GHB)	50 mg/kg body weight, divided into three daily doses	GABAA agonist GHB antagonist			5

Contd...

Medication	Dosage	Mechanism of action and target receptors	Pathways	Drug indication	*References
Memantlne	Tablet : 5 - 10 mg The recommended starting dose of Memantlne hydrochloride tablet is 5 mg once daily. The dose should be increased in 5 mg increments to 10 mg/day (5 mg twice daily), 15 mg/day (5 mg and 10 mg as separate doses), and 20 mg/day (10 mg twice daily). The minimum recommended interval between dose increases is one week.	n-methyl d-aspartate (NMDA) antagonist	glutamate	FDA approved drug Used as co-morbid therapy for antidepressant and alcoholism. Reduces alcohol consumption.	5 & 24
Acamprosate	Delayed release tablet : 333 mg/day	NMDA antagonist metabotropic glutamate receptor-5 (mGluR5) antagonist		Prescribed drug: FDA approved drug, reduces symptoms of protracted abstinence associated with chronic alcohol exposure and alcohol withdrawal	5 & 6
Disulfiram	Tablet: 400 mg/day for the first week and 200 mg/day as maintenance	acetaldehyde dehydrogenase inhibition	alcohol metabolism	FDA approved drug. When taken in combination with alcohol, Disulfiram causes aldehyde formation by physical reactions, which causes nausea, flushing, and heart palpitations The knowledge that such a reaction is likely if alcohol is consumed acts as a deterrent to drinking	5,6 & 15

Contd...

Medication	Dosage	Mechanism of action and target receptors	Pathways	Drug indication	*References
Vareniclne	Tablet: 1mg twice daily along with combination therapy and / or therapy for co-morbid condition for heavy drinker	α4β2 partial agonist		FDA approved drug for smoking secession: Used in co-morbid disorders like tobacco consumer and alcohol dependency for heavy drinker	5,25, & 26
Prazosin	Short half-life of 2 to 3 hours and duration of action of 6 to 10 hours. Therefore, its use is limited to 2 or 3 times daily dosing. Higher (30 to 50 mg) and more frequent (2 to 3 times per day) dosages might be needed because of the drug's short half-life.	α1 antagonist	adrenergic	FDA approved drug used for high blood pressure and Benign Prostatic Hyperplasia (BPH). Used for Combination therapy to treat alcoholism	5 & 27

References from 5 to 27 are from Table 1.

ALCOHOL WITHDRAWAL SYMPTOMS

Alcohol withdrawal condition is when an alcoholic reduces and completely stop drinking abruptly. Several features are observable along with the withdrawal symptoms especially significant distress, impairment psychosocial behaviour, occupational anomaly and several other remarkable symptoms. Withdrawal symptoms of alcohol dependency encompass serious medical consequences, if not monitored or supervised by medical practitioners. Withdrawal of alcohol indicates addictive disease and should not be neglected. Alcohol withdrawal symptoms can begin as early as two hours after the last drink, persist for weeks, and range from mild anxiety and shakiness to severe complications, such as seizures and Delirium Tremens (also called DTs). The death rates from DTs are estimated to range from 1% to 5%. Out of alcoholic population, it has been observed the most intense and serious syndrome associated with AW. DT is characterized by confusion, hyperthermia (fever), severe agitation, tremor, disorientation, persistent hallucinations, and large increases in heart rate, breathing rate, pulse, and blood pressure.[28] The other common factors with alcohol withdrawal symptoms incorporate: (i) Convulsions and/or tremors; (ii) Cold sweating (iii) Anxiety & irritation; (iv) Vomiting; (v) Nausea; (vi) Seizures; (vii) Hallucinations; (viii) Diaphoresis; and (ix) Insomnia.[29 & 30] Alcohol dependency results many severe disorders in the body system, therefore, overall vital signs and symptoms for physical examination at the time of AW and during the treatment of AW should be considered viz. continuous monitoring for arrhythmia, heart functions, blood pressure, congestive heart failure, alcoholic hepatitis, cirrhosis, alcoholic pancreatitis, infectious diseases like tuberculosis, haemorrhagic disorders in Gastrointestinal system and nervous system impairment. Blood pressure and heartbeat should be stabilized and should be balanced by injectable IV fluids and nutritional balance.[28]

1.2 ALCOHOL WITHDRAWAL SYNDROME (AWS)

Recently Sodium Oxybate, a physiological neurotransmitter derived from GABA has been approved for AWS and relapse. The safely and efficacy has been established in reducing the anxiety and depression associated with AWS. New approaches for the treatment of alcohol dependency are emerging for reduction of alcohol intake. In this regard Nalmefene is an μ- and α-opioid receptor antagonist and □-opioid partial agonist, which has been suggested with reduction of alcohol in heavy drinker.[31] Naltrexone and Acamprosate are also given for continuous abstinence therapy. Health practitioner has to decide which drug is more effective by observing response and monitoring by required lab tests of the patient; however, changing drug often creates discomfort to the patient. Therefore, the same drug continuing treatment may help in establishing “therapeutic alliance” between patients and health practitioner, which helps in achieving favourable results.

DETOXIFICATION

Detoxification is defined as the medical procedure for rapidly and safely achieving alcohol free state in a subject with alcohol dependency. Alcohol detoxification has more health risks associated than the other drug dependencies. The overall health condition should be considered, whether the patient needs to be treated in outpatient or inpatient management setup for detoxification. Patient disposing mild to moderate AW symptoms, can be considered for **outpatient treatment** management. Patient reflecting no medical conditions or severe psychiatric disorders (history of AW seizures or DT's) can complicate the withdrawal process. In addition, candidates for outpatient detoxification should have a sober significant presentation and come along with a reliable support person. Ambulatory AW patients should report to their treatment centre daily so that the clinician can reassess the patient's symptoms, the occurrence of medical complications, and ongoing treatment effectiveness. The factors to be considered for hospitalization or **inpatient treatment** to manage detoxification which includes history of significant AW symptoms, high levels of recent drinking, a history of withdrawal seizures or DT's, and the co-occurrence of a serious medical or psychiatric illness.[28] Abrupt stopping of alcohol consumption results DT. Addicted patients or long term drinkers are at more risk and could be fatal or result in coma if not monitored under medical environment. Medically managed withdrawal or detoxification is the very first step in recovery of patient. Diazepam (20-60 mg/day), or Chlordiazepoxide (50-150 mg/day), Thiamine 50 mg/3 times a day tablets or 100 mgs are found to be more effective therapies for detoxification.[32]

COMBINATION OR ADJUNCT THERAPY

The most effective strategy for alcohol treatment is combination therapy, because of the interaction among neurotransmitters and combination of therapeutic agents. Combination of Naltrexone and Acamprosate is found to be more effective in relapse of alcoholism. Acamprosate and concurrent psychosocial therapy revealed enhancement in duration of abstinence, however, with little impact of craving. Naltrexone with medication management versus cognitive-behavioural intervention demonstrated reduction in heavy drinking pattern. Along with supportive psychotherapy Naltrexone revealed increased abstinence. Outcome of opioid antagonist and integrated psychosocial treatment were significantly noted higher than the monotherapy for alcoholism. Improving overall health by treatment for mental health disorders improves self esteem of individual which impact on abstinence. Antidepressants showed no major role in treating alcoholism, however, patients overcome by depression due to alcohol dependency, hence improve the abstinence.[10]

PSYCHOPHARMACOTHERAPIES

Psychopharmacotherapy approaches are cumulative efforts to deal with the alcoholism and psychiatric disorders in all age groups. More emphasis is given on anticraving medication and alcohol abuse intervention. Due to alcohol consumption the brain neurotransmitters gets affected including dopamine, gamma-amino butyric acid (GABA), glutamate, serotonin, adenosine, norepinephrine and opiods peptides and their receptors. The dopaminergic pathways are mediated by alcohol consumption, which gives pleasurable and stimulant effects from the ventral segmental area to the nucleus accumbency. Hence, repeated consumption results dependency. Researchers have targeted this dopamine system which may reduce the reinforcement effects of alcohol and thereby reduce dependency. Realisation is also a common problem with alcohol dependency; therefore, anticraving medication therapy has always been focus since yester years. In Table 1, compilation of anticraving drugs is summarised for ready reference. **Agonist** is a substance, which combines with the cell receptor to produce some reaction that is typical for that substance. On the other hand, **antagonist** is a chemical, which opposes or reduces the action.

2.1 Opiate antagonist: Opiate peptides are class of neurotransmitters that binds to opioid receptors in the brain. Opioids mimic the effect of these opiate peptides. Activity and production of Opiate peptides appear to be affected by alcohol consumption; hence, the medication which blocks the opioid activity may block the craving for alcohol. Several μ-opioid agonists are more effective for alcohol dependency. Several opioid agonists are discussed in Table 1 used for medication for alcoholism.

2.2 Glutamate antagonist: Physiological craving by targeting NMDA receptor (*N*-methyl-D-aspartate receptor) has been found to reduce craving for alcohol. Some Glutamate antagonists are demonstrated in Table 1.

2.3 Serotonergic medication: Serotonin is a monoamine neurotransmitter which regulates the diverse physiological functions, including body rhythms, sleep, mood states, appetite, and consumatory behaviour. Serotonin receptor functions are altered by alcohol consumption by stimulating Dopaminergic activity, which produces the rewarding effects of alcohol. Many studies revealed that increasing levels of serotonin helped significant improvement in abstinence efforts (Table 1).

2.4 Dopamine antagonists: Most antipsychotics are dopamine antagonists. They have been found useful in treating schizophrenia, bipolar disorder, and stimulant psychosis. Several other dopamine antagonists are antiemetics used in the treatment of nausea and vomiting (Table 1).

Psychopharmacology and Co-morbidity psychiatric disorders:

Co-morbid condition is presence of two or more psychiatric disorders at a time in which one is substance dependency like alcohol or drugs and other may be mental illness. When a patient is suffering from two or more mental disorder of same group of diagnosis is referred as **homotypic co-morbidity** (*e.g.* Cannabis and Alcohol). When a patient is suffering from two or more different mental disorder in which one is substance dependency is referred as **heterotypic co-morbidity** (*e.g.* Depression and Alcohol).[33] To understand the pharmacological and behavioural treatment with co-morbid psychiatric disorders, there are several clinical issues need to be demonstrated. (i) Whether the FDA approved medicine for psychotropic medications are effective for alcohol dependency as well (ii) Whether the pharmacological and behavioural treatment of alcoholics diverge from non co-morbid alcoholics (iii) Whether positive results are not found in the treatment of other disorders for alcoholism or for the psychiatric disorder (iv) Whether the treatment for alcohol dependency and psychiatric condition should be conducted simultaneously or consecutively (v) Whether the treatment strategy differ for each type of psychiatric co-morbidity. Researchers have focus more on four major psychiatric disorders viz. Depression, anxiety, bipolar disorder and schizophrenia.[34] Several studies are published every year to delineate the most effective strategies for the treatment of co-morbid psychiatric condition in alcoholics. The review of literature on co-occurrence of psychiatric disorders reveals on pharmacological agents or psychosocial treatments treated along with psychiatric disorder medication; however, the effectiveness of co-treatment is still underway to guide the treatment for such population.

DEPRESSION

Depression and alcoholism is a complex association because of overlapping symptoms like neurobiological abnormalities and similar treatments (pharmacological and psychosocial). Two classes of **Antidepressants**—(i) **the Selective Serotonin Reuptake Inhibitors** (SSRIs), which affect the production and/or absorption of the neurotransmitter serotonin have been evaluated in patients with co-morbid depression and alcohol use. These antidepressant has shown better results in managing depression and alcohol dependency (Imipramine, Desipramine and Nefazodone); (ii) **Tricyclic antidepressants** (TCAs) showed no positive results for selective serotonin reuptake inhibitors in some studies (Sertraline, Fluoxetine, Citalopram). The TCAs, including Desipramine and Imipramine, have been found effective in treating depression in alcoholics, but there is no consistent evidence that they are effective in decreasing alcohol consumption. With these mixed results and considering the potential for overdose, the use of TCAs in alcohol-abusing patients may be unwise.[35] Few studied indicates sertraline would be the best choice for moderate – to severe anti depression, because of the efficacy, acceptability and lower cost. However, as per WHO list Fluoxetine and Amitriptyline among the antidepressants are approved in essential drug list which limits the drug of choice.[32, 36, 37, 38 & 39]

ANTICRAVING AGENTS

3.2.1 Acamprosate: It is an FDA approved drug, it is widely available in US and Europe. It is an N-methyl-D-aspartate (NMDA) receptor antagonist for the brain chemical (*i.e.*, neurotransmitter) Glutamate. The mechanism of action is still not know, however, it has been estimated that Acamprosate affects calcium channels with subsequent decrease in activity of excitatory system in the CNS. Interactions with other receptors are currently being studied. Acamprosate showed positive results in meta-analysis for co-morbid condition, however, could not cure the symptoms of primary depression. Other studies have indicated that Acamprosate may be helpful in achieving abstinence, at least partially by fading withdrawal symptoms in long term alcohol users by recovering chemical balance in the brain.[40] Acamprosate is recommended for the patients who goals for complete abstinence, thus can be used in combination therapy, and can be supervised medically for withdrawal. It can be used safely with other neuropsychiatric therapy. The effectiveness of this drug is observed in 5 to 8 days and the therapy can be continued even if the patient relapses to alcohol use. This drug is more useful in the patients who are already challenged with liver derangements and are treated with opioid for pain or addiction because the drug is excreted through renal channel and does not give negative effects to endogenous or exogenous opioid. This fact advocates the use of drug in combination therapy safely. Additional studies will help to answer questions about the use of Acamprosate in alcoholism treatment for co-morbid psychiatric treatment approach. Research establishing its efficacy was conducted in patients without co-morbid psychiatric disorders.[42] Many clinical trials registered on primary registry are being completed and few are undergoing to demonstrate the effectiveness of Acamprosate for detoxification in alcohol dependent therapeutic regime and co-morbid psychiatric disorder such as bipolar and depression. Combination therapy with other compounds/drugs such as Gabapentin, Naltrexone etc. for treatment of psychiatric disorders and to follow-up the detoxification regime are also being studied and few trials are ongoing.[43]

3.2.2 Disulfiram: Disulfiram has been approved by US FDA. This is the first medicine used for the treatment of alcohol dependency, which dampen the craving by producing unpleasant physiological reaction along with alcohol consumption, hence act as anticraving and self control in the patient. It is an evidence-based prevention therapy used in the management of alcohol-use disorders and may promote total abstinence.[44 & 45] It has been suggested that the drug should be used or avoided in the patients with liver dysfunction, but it may be useful for other groups.[46] Not much studies have been conducted to prove effectiveness of Disulfiram alone for alcoholic depression. However, there are many studies reported with combination therapy of Disulfiram for the treatment of other substance dependency, such as cocaine. Also combination with other compounds like Lorazepam for co-morbid anxiety disorder, and in treatment of other psychiatric disorders and also in managing the HIV patients shown significant results.[47] It may also help in medication after detoxification for alcohol dependency and depression by maintaining abstinence. Disulfiram is not enlisted in WHO essential list of drugs. Disulfiram metabolise in the body and produces acetaldehyde which is highly toxic, and patient has aversive reaction like vomiting, flushing, headache and severe anxiety. Therefore, the person develops reversal for alcohol and stops completely if given in prescribed form and under proper supervision of healthcare practitioner. However, some people may tolerate these effects and some may quit from the therapy, which makes Disulfiram not a successful drug of choice.[42]

3.2.3 Naltrexone: Naltrexone, approved by the FDA for the treatment of alcoholism, which blocks action of opioid, hence it is an opioid antagonist. Additionally, Naltrexone is non-selective opioid antagonist with high affinity for the μ-opioid receptor and to some extend for the μ-opioid receptor. Due to prolonged exposure of alcohol the μ-opioid receptors are up-regulated; therefore, remarkable therapeutic results are achieved. As increased activity of μ-opioid receptors may induce depression/dysphoria by alcohol withdrawal. As a result reduction in frequency of consumption and decline in per consumption is achieved.[48] Some clinical trials suggests that Naltrexone can be used as adjunct therapy for alcohol detoxification and psychotherapy, therefore, may be used for prevention of relapse in alcoholic dependency. It also reflects psychosocial mechanism in patients of self administration in retrospective studies. It reduces craving and increase abstinence, it hinders the initial drink reinforcement resulting adversity towards alcohol dependency even in heavy drinker. Because of its moderate effects Naltrexone if better choice of drug to the patients as compare to Disulfiram, because they know that drinking is not completely prohibited along with the management of treatment with Naltrexone. Studies have shown the positive effects on major psychiatric illnesses, including schizophrenia, bipolar disorder, schizoaffective disorder, and co-morbid alcohol dependence. Naltrexone can have a good clinical response as measured by treatment retention and alcohol consumption.[49] In other study, the results showed that Naltrexone treated patients reported lower levels of alcohol craving, fewer drinks consumed per occasion, fewer drinking days, and lower rates of relapse to heavy drinking compared with placebo-treated patients.[42] There are very many clinical trials that are being registered on primary registry about the safety and efficacy of Naltrexone and also with combination therapy for various co-morbid psychiatric patient suffering from alcoholism in care in inpatient care. Naltrexone is also being studied with combination of other pharmacotherapeutic compounds for studied for alcoholism.[50]

3.3 Anti-anxiety Treatment: Medication which is well known for treatment for anxiety disorders include Benzodiazepines; TCAs; SSRIs; and other serotonergic medications (*i.e.*, medications that affect serotonin receptors), such as Buspirone, Benzodiazepines are widely used for anxiety disorders, but some of their properties make their use controversial in patients with co-morbid alcohol use disorders and anxiety disorders. Benzodiazepine is not drug of choice for co-morbid condition as dependency for Benzodiazepine is again need proper medication for its motor and cognitive impairment associated with alcohol use.[42] Both TCAs and SSRIs have been found effective in treating anxiety disorders, but their use in dually diagnosed patients has not been formally investigated. The SSRIs often are the first line of treatment for anxiety disorders because of their relatively minor side effects. Given recent evidence of their efficacy in treating alcohol use and depressive symptoms in dually diagnosed in patients, further study of these medications in this population need to be studied.[51 & 52]

Post-Traumatic Stress Disorder (PTSD) is the most frequently occurring anxiety disorder (*i.e.*, compared with generalized anxiety disorder (GAD) and panic disorder, affecting 5.6 percent of respondents diagnosed as alcohol abusers. Other medications used for PTSD patients include the monoamine oxidase inhibitors (MAOIs) and anticonvulsants. MAOIs should be used with caution. It is imperative that patients taking these medications avoid foods and beverages containing the chemical tyramine— for example, beer on tap, red wines, liqueurs, overly ripe foods, salami, and aged cheeses. Patients actively abusing alcohol may be unable to adhere to this dietary restriction because of impaired judgment. The anticonvulsants are more promising because there are some evidence that they may be effective in treating anxiety disorders. Buspirone a serotonergic drug has been formally evaluated in patients with co-morbid generalized anxiety disorder and alcohol dependence. Although several of these clinical studies suggested that buspirone reduced anxiety symptoms and reduction in alcohol use, other studies reported that it had no effect in reducing anxiety or alcohol use. These mixed results have left clinicians appropriately skeptical about the utility of this medication in this population.[53]

3.4 Anti-psychotic Medications: The first line of treatment for patients with schizophrenia or psychotic disorders is antipsychotic or neuroleptic medications. Acute psychosis restrict a person to participate in social, community, and treatment activities, therefore, focus of treatment should be to stabilizing these symptoms. There are several classes of antipsychotic drugs with differing pharmacology, side effects, and receptor-binding affinity. However, no sufficient evidences are available to prove that one type of antipsychotic is superior in treating the dually diagnosed patient. Based on the mechanisms of action, of the different classes of antipsychotics, the underlying psychology and neurobiology of the disorders, and clinical experience some general actions are known to suggest positive results. The newer antipsychotics have been reported to better treat negative symptoms and have fewer movement disorder side effects (*e.g.*, muscle spasms). Because negative symptoms may play a role in the aetiology or maintenance of substance use disorders therefore, people may use alcohol or other drugs to self-medicate the negative symptoms.[42] Schizophrenia is a chronic, relapsing disorder, with symptoms beginning in late adolescence or early adulthood. The symptoms are hallucinations and delusions, by apathy, avolition, anhedonia, and disorganized thinking or behaviour. Clozapine may be effective in reducing symptoms of alcohol use disorders and schizophrenia in dually diagnosed patients.[54] Antipsychotic medication including potent blockers of the dopamine D2 receptor are often used for treatment for such population. Novel antipsychotic agent Quetiapine may reduce stimulant craving in co-morbid patients.[55]

Emerging Pharmacotherapies:

Effective strategies to treat alcohol dependency are required through novel drug innovations and management strategies. The strategies may depend on the health condition, psychiatric disorder and severity of the psychiatric condition. There are many potential pharmacological medications for alcohol and other substance dependency and are being used currently; however, not many medications are approved for human use because of their limited beneficiary effects. Hence, there is a considerable requirement at present to address the alcoholism and other substance dependency.

Emerging pharmacotherapies treatment model and management for alcoholic patients are suggested to be considered on the grounds –

1. The patient is adoptive towards treatment;
2. The stage of alcoholism and/or change of situation;
3. The potential for relapse;
4. The severity of ongoing combination therapy including psychiatric disorders;
5. Tolerability of patient for treatment; and
6. Pregnant patient medication.

For heavy drinker the clinician should decide the abstinence is the interim goal and revise the goal as the patients adopt the treatment. Maintaining the complete abstinence is the safer strategy for long term success.[6]

Newer approaches are focussing on controlling craving for alcohol intake, where craving means the neurobiological adaption of the gratification circuits induced by alcohol. It has been suggested that specific pharmacological therapy for the three subtypes of craving defined by psychobiological model for reduction in alcohol consumption are in focus. In particular, they suggested Naltrexone and Sodium Oxybate for reward craving;

Acamprosate, Baclofen and Sodium Oxybate for relief craving; and an SSRI, Baclofen, Topiramate and Ondansetron for obsessive craving.[56] However, Naltrexone oral and injection (380 mg) for therapeutic plasma release has been approved by FDA with black-box warning for liver toxicity. Injectable preparation provides effective results in heavy drinkers. Its effects lasts for four weeks which retain abstinence in alcoholics during that period.[57] Nalmefene is better drug of choice as compared to Naltrexone as it has longer half-life central opioid receptors and lower liver toxicity. This suggestive to use before starting the alcohol consumption means targeted use of drug before 1-2 hours prior to the anticipated time of drinking, or as soon as possible if the patient has already started drinking.[58] Several clinical trials are being registered on primary registries of national and international levels with different pharmacotherapeutic approaches which are clubbed with psychopharmacotherapeutic treatment management. Recently, in HIV patients the effects of Topiramate on heavy drinkers are tested.[18 & 59]

In alcohol withdrawal symptoms, Gabapentin has shown superior results than Naltrexone in terms of achieving longer abstinence. This is experimentation towards evaluating combinations of therapeutics that enhance treatment efficacy. In this specific study Gabapentin was added to Naltrexone to treat insomnia and mood instability. The results supported the hypothesis and in addition improved drinking outcomes.[60] Recently, few medication candidates have been abandoned for reasons of side effects (Rimonaband) or lack of efficacy (Aripiprasole).[61] Prazosin is and adrenergic receptor antagonist which is given for the treatment of trauma, nightmares and sleep disturbance, at the dose of 16 mg versus placebo. Trial is undergoing in reducing alcohol consumption and decreasing symptoms of post traumatic stress disorder in alcoholic patients.[62] Citalopram in patients who were moderate or less drinker or initial starters showed decrease in drinking behaviour in clinical trials, however, in heavy drinker showed trend in opposite direction. Therefore, the studies are ongoing to establish the useful effects of Citalopram in heavy drinkers.[63] There are several other compounds which are in early stage of drug development as novel target for alcohol dependency and psychological disorders viz., Ibudilast (a neuroimmune modulator that inhibits phosphodiestrase-4a and 10); Ketamine (antidepressant properties) shows good response in family history of alcoholics, however, co-morbid use is still in trial. All these compound information can be reviewed from primary registries.[18]

CONCLUSION

Reduction in alcohol consumption could be considered as valid interim goal for any therapeutic approach. From analysis of literature to decipher the most effective treatment for alcoholism remains a challenge for researchers and also for clinicians. Interdisciplinary efforts are been made to reduce the knowledge gaps to explain the brain's neurotransmission and the behaviour pattern of addiction of alcoholics. As prevalence of psychiatric co-morbidity significantly high in alcoholic population with juxtaposed depression, anxiety, bipolar disorder, schizophrenia, therefore, concomitant therapy of Pharmacotherapy and Psychopharmacotherapy approach is adopted by the clinicians who posses unique expertise for such treatment for better results. An effort has been made to compile the most updated Pharmacotherapies currently adopted also explain the co-morbid complications in fewer studies. However, co-morbid psychiatric disorders still remains a big challenge to address the most effective treatment for alcoholism. Novel approaches to treat alcoholism (with neurological disorders and psychosocial disorders) are being focusing more on anticraving and prevention of relapse. Efforts are being made to delineate most effective dosage regimen for detoxification. In some developed countries like United States and Europe Topiramate, Baclofen and Gabapentin are used as off-label drugs. Although tremendous advances by the researchers and clinicians has been made; however, more effective future therapies with more precise dosage regimen in pharmacotherapy, combination therapies and for co-morbid disorders are need of hour to get rid of this psychosocial problem from the society.

REFERENCES AND NOTES

1. World Health Organization; Alcohol and Injury in Emergency Department: **2002**
2. R. Room, D. Jernigen, and Carlini-Marlatt. Alcohol in Developing Societies. Finnish Foundation for Alcohol Studies, Helsinki, Finland. **2002**
3. Griffith Edwards and Milton M. Gross. Alcohol dependence-Provisional description of a clinical syndrome. British Medical Journal, **1976**, 1, 1058-1061.
4. World Health Organisation. Classification of Mental & Behavioral Disorders: Diagnostic Criteria for Research Guidelines, WHO-Geneva. **1992.**

5. Carolina *et.al.* Pharmacological Approaches to Reducing Craving in Patients with Alcohol Use Disorders, *CNS Drugs*, **2014**, 26 (4), 343-360.
6. Use of Pharmacotherapies in the treatment of alcohol use disorders and opioid dependency in primary care. BioMed Research International; Article ID 137020. **2015**.
7. N. Ryder, W. Cullen, J. Barry, G. Bury, E. Keenan, B.P. Smyth. Prevalence of problem alcohol use among patients attending primary care for methadone treatment. *BMC Fam. Pract.* **2009**, 10, 42..
8. François aille and Hervé Martini. Nalmefene: a new approach to the treatment of alcohol dependence. *Subst Abuse Rehabil.* **2014**, 5, 87–94.
9. S.H. Williams. Medications for Treating Alcohol Dependence. *Am Fam Physician.* **2005**, 72(9), 1775-1780.
10. J.G. Modell, J.M. Mountz, F.B. Glaser, J.Y. Lee. Effect of Haloperidol on measures of craving and impaired control in alcoholic subjects. *Alcohol Clin Exp Res.* **1993**, 17(2), 234–40.
11. Zhongshu Yang and Glen L Xiong Alcohol-Related Psychosis Treatment & Management; Updated: Dec 03, **2015**. http://emedicine.medscape.com/article/289848-treatment
12. Martinotti G, Di Nicola M, Janiri L. Efficacy and safety of Aripiprazole in alcohol dependence. American Journal of Drug and Alcohol Abuse. **2007**; 33(3): 393-401.
13. https://clinicaltrials.gov/ct2/show/NCT00561587?term=Quetiapine+AND+alcohol&rank=3 (last seen on 1 May 2017).
14. https://clinicaltrials.gov/ct2/show/NCT00746785?term=new+pharmacotherapy+and+alcohol&rank=1 (last seen on 7 May 2017).
15. G. Addolorato, A. Armuzzi, G. Gasbarrini. Pharmacological approaches to the management of alcohol addiction & Alcoholism. Treatment Study Group. European Review for Medical and Pharmacological Sciences, **2002**; 6: 89-97.
16. R.J. Dougherty, R.R. Gates. The role of buspirone in the management of alcohol withdrawal: a preliminary investigation. J Subst Abuse Treat. **1990**;7(3):189-92.
17. Gregory B. Collins, Mark S. Mcallister, Kamala Adur. Drug adjuncts for treating alcohol dependence. Cleveland Clinic Journal of Medicine. Vol. 73, No. 7. July, **2006.**
18. K.A. Michalak And Grazyna Biala. Alcohol Dependence Neurobiology And Treatment. *Acta Poloniae Pharmaceutica ñ Drug Research*, **2015**, 73(1), 312.

19. V. Vengeliene, C.A. Heidbreder, R. Spanagel. The effects of lamotrigine on alcohol seeking and relapse. Neuropharmacology. **2007** Dec; 53(8):951-7.

20. C. Richter, *et.al.* Levetiracetam for the treatment of alcohol withdrawal syndrome: a multicenter, prospective, randomized, placebo-controlled trial. *Clin Psychopharmacol.* **2010**, 30(6), 720-5.

21. G. Rubio, *et.al.* Effects of Zonisamide in the treatment of alcohol dependence. Clin Neuropharmacol. **2010** Sep-Oct;33(5):250-3. doi: 10.1097/WNF.0b013e3181f0ed9a.

22. Jia Liu, Lu-Ning Wang. Baclofen for alcohol withdrawal. First published: 28 February **2013** Editorial Group: Cochrane Drugs and Alcohol Group DOI: 10.1002/14651858.CD008502.pub3.

23. Agnieszka Michalak and Grazyna Biala. Alcohol Dependence – Neurobiology and Treatment. Acta Pol Pharm. **2016** Jan-Feb;73(1):3-12.

24. Future Research Needs for First and second Generation Antipsychotics for Children and Young Adults. (https://www.ncbi.nlm.nih.gov/books/NBK84656/ (last seen on 27 May, **2017**).

25. Sandy Naegele. Varenicline for Alcohol Use Disorder. PGY1 Pharmacy Resident Central Texas Veterans Health Care System. The University of Texas at Austin College of Pharmacy. October 25, **2013**. http://sites.utexas.edu/pharmacotherapy-rounds/files/2015/09/naegele10-25-13.pdf.

26. Lara A. Ray, *et.al.* Varenicline, low dose Naltrexone, and their combination for heavy-drinking smokers: Human laboratory findings. Psychopharmacology (Berl). **2014** October; 231(19): 3843–3853. doi:10.1007/s00213-014-3519-0.

27. Prazosin for Alcohol Dependence and Posttraumatic Stress Disorder. **2012**. https://clinicaltrials.gov/ct2/show/record/NCT01518972.

28. Hugh Myrick, and Raymond F. Anton. Treatment of Alcohol Withdrawal. Alcohol Health & Research World. Vol. 22, No. 1, **1998**.

29. G.F. Koob, A.J. Roberts, G. Schulteis, *et.al.* Neurocircuitry targets in ethanol reward and dependence. *Alcohol Clin. Exp. Res*. **1998**;22:39.

30. Mayo-Smith MF. Pharmacological management of alcohol withdrawal. A meta-analysis and evidence-based practice guideline. American Society of Addiction Medicine Working Group on Pharmacological Management of Alcohol Withdrawal. *JAMA*, **1997**, 278, 144–5.

31. Fabio Caputo and Mauro Bernard. Alcoholism & Drug Dependence: New and Old drugs Treat Alcohol Use Disorders. *J. Alcohol Drug Depend.* **2014**, 2:3

32. N.G. Desai, R. Kumar, S.N. Sengupta, P. Sharma. Clinical Practice Guidelines for treatment of alcohol dependence. **2006**. (http://www.indianjpsychiatry.org/cpg/cpg2006/CPG-mgmt_14.pdf).
33. Vivek Kumar, Pankaj Kumar, M.S. Bhatia, Anurag Jhanjee. Substance abuse and Co-morbidity *Delhi Psychiatry J.*, **2010**, 13(1), 36-42.
34. Charlene E. Le Fauve, Raye Z. Litten, Carrie L. Randall et. al. Pharmacological Treatment of alcohol Abuse/Dependence with Psychiatric Co-morbidity. *Alcohol Clin. Exp. Res.* **2004**, 28(2), 302-312.
35. H.R. Kranzler, B.J. Rounsaville, eds. Dual Diagnosis and Treatment. New York: Marcel Dekker, **1998**.
36. N. Iovieno, *et.al.* Antidepressants for major depressive disorder and dysthymic disorder in patients with co-morbid alcohol use disorders: a meta- analysis of placebo-controlled randomized trials. J. Clin. Psychiatry. **2011**, 72(8), 1144–51.
37. Nunes EV, Levin FR. Treatment of depression in patients with alcohol or other drug dependence: a meta-analysis. JAMA. **2004**, 291(15), 1887–96.
38. WHO model list of essential medicines. 19th list (April 2015). Geneva: World Health Organization. **2015** (http://www.who.int/medicines/publications/essentialmedicines/EML_2015_FINAL_amended_NOV2015.pdf?ua=1, accessed 8 December 2016).
39. Yatan Pal Singh Balhara *et.al.* Co-occurring depression and alcohol-use disorders in South-East Asia: A narrative review. WHO South East Asia Journal of Public Health. April **2017**, (6)1.
40. B.J. Mason, R.L. Ownby. Acamprosate for the treatment of alcohol dependence: A review of double-blind, placebo-controlled trials. *CNS Spectrums*. **2000,** 5(2), 58–69.
41. D.E. Jonas, H.R. Amick, C. Feltner *et.al.* Pharmacotherapy for adults with alcohol use disorders in outpatient settings: a systematic review and meta-analysis. *J. Am. Med. Association*, **2014**, 311(18), 1889–1900.
42. L. Petrakis, *et.al.* Co-morbidity of Alcoholism and Psychiatric Disorders : An Overview: Ismene Alcohol Research and Health; **2002**. Vol. 26,No2, 81-89
43. https://clinicaltrials.gov/ct2/results?term=Acamprosate+and+alcohol&Search=Search. (last searched on 2 May 2017).
44. S. R¨osner, A. Hackl-Herrwerth, S. Leucht, P. Lehert, S. Vecchi, and M. Soyka. Acamprosate for alcohol dependence. Cochrane Database Systematic Reviews, Vol. 9, **2010**.
45. B. J. Mason, A. M. Goodman, S. Chabac, and P. Lehert. Effect of oral Acamprosate on abstinence in patients with alcohol dependence in a double-blind, placebo-controlled trial: the role of patient motivation. *Journal of Psychiatric Research*, **2006**, 40(5), 383–393.

46. Substance Abuse and Mental Health Services Administration, Medication-Assisted Treatment for Opioid Addiction in Opioid Treatment Programs A Treatment Improvement Protocol, HHS Publication no (SMA) 05-4058, TIP 43, **2007**).
47. https://clinicaltrials.gov/ct2/results?term=disulfiram+and+alcohol&Search=Search (last seen on 5 May 2017).
48. M.F. Olive. Pharmacotherapies for alcoholism: the old and the new. *CNS Neurol. Disord. Drug Targets*, **2010**, 9, 2.
49. S. Maxwell, M.S. Shinderman. Use of Naltrexone in the treatment of alcohol use disorders in patients with concomitant major mental illness. *J. Addictive Diseases*, **2000**, 19(3), 61–69.
50. https://clinicaltrials.gov/ct2/results?term=Naltrexone+and+alcohol&Search=Search, (last seen on 2 May 2017).
51. J.R. Cornelius, I.M. Salloum, M.D. Cornelius *et.al.* Preliminary report: Double-blind, placebo-controlled study of Fluoxetine in depressed alcoholics. *Psychopharmacology Bulletin* **1995** 31(2), 297–303.
52. J.R. Cornelius, I.M. Salloum, J.G. Ehler, et. al. Fluoxetine in depressed alcoholics: A double- blind, placebo-controlled trial. *Archives of General Psychiatry*, 54(8):700–705, **1997a**.
53. H. Myrick, K.T. Brady, R. Malcolm. New developments in the pharmacotherapy of alcohol dependence. American Journal on Addictions. 10(Suppl.) pp. 3–15, **2001.**
54. R.E. Drake, H. Xie, G.J. Mchugo, A.I. Green. Effects of Clozapine on alcohol and drug use disorders among patients with schizophrenia. Schizophrenia Bulletin, 26(2):441–449, **2000.**
55. E.S. Brown, V.A. Nejtek, D.C. Perantie, L. Bobadilla. Quetiapine in bipolar disorder and cocaine dependence. Bipolar Disord. **2002**. 4(6), 406 –11). (Main Ref. Pharmacological treatment of alcohol Abuse/Dependence with co-morbid condition. Alcoholism: Clinical and Experimental Research, Vol. 28, No. 2, February **2004).**
56. G. Fertonani Affini, *et.al.* New therapeutic approaches in alcohol dependence: reduction of consumption as a step in the therapeutic goal; *Journal of Psychopathology*, **2013**, 19, 164-171.
57. Agnieszka Michalak And Grazyna Biala. Alcohol Dependence Neurobiology And Treatment. Acta Poloniae Pharmaceutica ñ Drug Research, Vol. 73 No. 1 pp. 312, **2015.**
58. EMA Available at http://www.ema.europa.eu/docs/en_GB/document_library/EPAR_Product _Information/human/002583/WC5001 40255.pdf [Last accessed 10 September, 2014.

59. Topiramate to Reduce Heavy Drinking in HIV-Positive Heavy Drinkers http://clinicaltrias.gov/show/NCT01764685 (last seen 27 June 2017)
60. R.F. Anton, *et.al.* Gabapentin combined with Naltrexone for the treatment of alcohol dependence. *Am J Psychiatry*, **2011**, 168:709-717.
61. J. Franck, N.J. Lindstrom. Pharmacotherapy for alcohol dependence: status of current treatments; *Current Opinion in Neurobiology*, **2013**, 23, 692–699.
62. Prazosin for Alcohol Dependence and Posttraumatic Stress Disorder (PTSD) https://clinicaltrials.gov/ct2/show/record/NCT01518972 (last seen on 5 May 2017).
63. Citalopram Effects on Craving and Dopamine Receptor Availability in Alcoholics https://clinicaltrials.gov/ct2/show/NCT01657760 (last seen on 5 May 2017).

Editors' Note

Alcoholism being a complex disorder requires additional psychological and psychiatric therapy besides drugs therapy. Psychopharmacotherapy approaches are cumulative efforts to deal with the alcoholism and psychiatric disorders. The understanding of basis and the recent advances in use of various Psychopharmacotherapy practices is required to treat the alcoholic patients. The combination therapy is most effective strategy for alcohol treatment because of the interaction among neurotransmitters and combination of therapeutic agents e.g. Combination of Naltrexone and Acamprosate is found to be more effective in relapse of alcoholism. Similar detailed clinical analysis of dual drugs combinations would provide better management of alcoholics.

❑❑❑

9

Substance Abuse Disorder and its Management

Gauri Shanker Kaloiya* and Mohit Kumar**

Abstract

There are a number of problems with 'substance dependence' that present to clinicians. To begin with, detoxification can become much more problematic. The variable pattern of intake, availability of diverse combinations, interaction of multiple etiological factors, and prevalent co morbidities make this group a heterogeneous one. In this chapter mainly we have focussed on substances that are taken in different patterns for different reasons. The combinations might 'feel different', 'feel better' or are used for self-medication and also focus on type of substance use and their dependencies and their psychological management.

Keywords: Substance, Disorder, Management

INTRODUCTION

Substance use disorders are a major cause of death and disability. Numerous clinical studies indicate that there is an association between substance use and personality disorders, with evidence that personality pathology may influence both the aetiology and course of substance use disorders.[1,2] The

* National Drug Dependence Treatment Centre, All India Institute of Medical Sciences (AIIMS) New Delhi.

** Department of Psychiatry, All India Institute of Medical Sciences (AIIMS) New Delhi.

definitions of substance abuse and dependence are based on the dependence syndrome of Griffith Edwards.[3] Substance abuse is a maladaptive pattern of substance use leading to significant adverse consequences manifested by psychosocial, medical, or legal problems or use in situations in which it is physically hazardous that must recur during a 12-month period. Since a diagnosis of substance dependence prompts a diagnosis of abuse, tolerance, withdrawal and compulsive use are generally not present in individuals with a diagnosis of substance abuse. Dependence is generally thought to indicate a central role of the substance in an individual's life, with problems relating to controlling intake, and the emergence of physical and psychological difficulties despite which the individual continues to use the substance. Substance dependence has been considered a more valid and reliable diagnosis than substance abuse.

Substance abuses are seen in both gender, all races and ethnic groups and in all socioeconomic strata. It does not discriminate by geographical location, race or religion. Whether it is alcohol, inhalants, pharmaceuticals or heroin, it can have the same tragic consequences: wasted lives, ruined families, and communication torn apart. The numbers are staggering. 6 to 20% of acute hospital admission is related to alcohol. Every ten second another person dies as a result of tobacco use. It has been seen that adolescents, young adults and children are the worst sufferers.

EPIDEMIOLOGY

Epidemiology is concerned with the distribution and determinants of substance intake occurrence. Epidemiology of substance use is more of social epidemiology as it focuses on subgroups and trends rather the population. A Department of Health and Human Services' (DHHS) survey in 2002 found that 56% of all admissions to treatment facilities were for multiple substances, and 68.9% were male, 90.0% were adults (18 years or older), with most falling between the ages of 25 and 44. Adolescents (those under 18 years of age) were almost twice as likely to be mono-drug abusers. Adults from 18 to 44 years old were slightly more likely to be poly drug abusers, while adults 45 and over were significantly more likely to be mono-drug abusers. In contrast, Chen & Kandel[4] found a tendency for poly drug abusers to be young, with initiation of illicit polydrug abuse being rare after age 20. Polydrug abuse was lowest for those over 40 years old and highest among those under 20. Furthermore, research has suggested that the incidence of polydrug abuse may decline with age.[5]

Of all admissions who reported alcohol abuse, 39.9% reported solely abusing alcohol compared to 60.1% who reported abusing alcohol along with some other substance. Similarly, 77.8% of the admissions reporting cocaine abuse and 79.9% of those using marijuana were polydrug abusers. Interestingly, higher proportions of polydrug abuse were seen among the lesser abused drugs; over 90% of sedative and hallucinogen abusers and about 80% of amphetamine and inhalant abusers reported polydrug abuse. National Institute on Drug Abuse (NIDA) survey found in 2001 and 2002 that more than 71% of the cocaine users represented multi drug episodes, as did approximately 53% of the heroin users, 74% of the marijuana users, and 54% of the methamphetamine users. The TEDS (Treatment Episode Data Set) data also indicated that roughly half of adolescents between the ages of 12 and 17 who were admitted for substance abuse treatment were being treated for a combination of both alcohol and marijuana. Among drug-involved death in 2001, the vast majority of deaths involved more than one drug, including cocaine (83%), heroin (89%), and methamphetamine (92%).

TYPE OF SAD

According to the mental health clinician's handbook, Diagnostic and Statistical Manual of Mental Disorders (DSM), fourth edition text revised (DSM IV-TR), all of the substances with the exceptions of nicotine and caffeine, have disorders of two types: substance use disorders and substance-induced disorders. Substance use disorders include abuse and dependence. Substance-induced disorders include intoxication, withdrawal, and various mental states (dementia, psychosis, anxiety, mood disorder, etc.) that the substance induces when it is used.[16]

List of Addictions to Substances

Substance use disorders in the DSM-IV-TR provide a list of addictions relating to the following substances:

- Alcohol
- Tobacco
- Opioids (like heroin)

- Prescription drugs (sedatives, hypnotics, or anxiolytics like sleeping pills and tranquilizers)
- Cocaine
- Cannabis (marijuana)
- Amphetamines (like methamphetamine, known as meth)
- Hallucinogens
- Inhalants
- Phencyclidine (known as PCP or Angeldust)
- Other unspecified substances

List of Impulse Control Disorders

The DSM-IV-TR lists disorders where impulses cannot be resisted, which could be considered a type of addiction. The following is a list of the recognized impulse control disorders:

- Intermittent explosive disorder (compulsive aggressive and assaultive acts)
- Kleptomania (compulsive stealing)
- Pyromania (compulsive setting of fires)
- Gambling

List of Addictions - Behavioral

It has been suggested one of the types of addictions is behavioral addiction. The following is a list of behaviors that have been noted to be addictive:

- Food (eating)
- Sex
- Pornography (attaining, viewing)
- Using computers/the internet
- Playing video games
- Working
- Exercising
- Spiritual obsession (as opposed to religious devotion)
- Pain (seeking)
- Cutting
- Shopping

ETIOLOGY

Theories

Cognitive Expectancy Theory

According to this theory substance additive behaviour are chosen over healthy behaviours due to human expectation. When a person who have taken substance expects the pros and cons of addictive behaviour favourably outweigh the pros and cons of healthy behaviour, they will choose addiction. For example someone might be mistakenly believe that healthier choices will lead to boredom. These expectations about substance addiction may develop by observing others. This can be through direct or indirect observation. For instance, a movie can interpret a drug dealer as someone who is sexually popular with a glamorous and exciting life. Once these expectations develop, they are often resistant to change.[6]

Social Learning Theory

According to this theory, based on observation of the person who is engaging in addictive substance use behaviour can lead to the increase of addiction. We often observe the behaviour and their reaction of other person using addictive substances, we always wish to repeat what we saw. For example when our parent come home with some agitation, exhausted from work, he or she take some substance like alcohol, then becomes relaxed and enjoying to be around. We conclude that alcohol is good way of coping with stress.[7]

Social Factors

The initiation of young people into the recreational substance abuse scene is complex of the most powerful predictors are social influences including behavior and attitudes of family and friends. Family influences such as parenting, permissive or tolerant attitudes and social influence like peer pressure have been implicated in substance use[8] but maintenance of such social behavior can be best understood by the 'problem behaviour' framework; it has been reported that young people begin with negative attitudes to Substance abuse, are exposed to drug users, acquire more positive attitudes, and then try the drugs.[10-11] Participation in underage drinking might bring adolescents into contact with a Substance-using environment in which they are more likely to be offered drugs, or increase their exposure to positive drug-related opinions and attitudes.

Family Factors

Family play an important role of substance abuse aside from genetic influence. Parent and older sibling taking substance serve as an important role model of substance taking behaviour in children. A person who did not live with both their natural parents were found to be at greater risk of substance use than those who came from an intact family. Overall, 60.6% of those from intact families used either cigarettes, alcohol or illicit drugs in some combination, compared to 67.9% of those from non-intact families. This difference was even more marked for cigarette smoking: 15.3% of adolescents from traditional, intact families smoked compared to 26.7% of those from non-traditional families. The picture was similar for regular alcohol and illicit drug use with 59.4% and 13.4% of those from intact families using these groups of substances, respectively, compared to 65.9% and 19.1% from non-intact families.[12]

Individual Factors

Adolescents and adults who use substances are less likely to be aware of negative consequences of use, have less negative attitudes about substances and more of positive outcome expectancies. Outcome expectancies represent intervening cognitive variables that connect memory and behavior, and reflect knowledge of a relationship between events and objects. Outcome expectancies, which are defined as the effects that individuals anticipate they would experience after taking substance.[9] These expectancies can be positive (*e.g.* 'Drinking alcohol can make parties more fun') or negative (*e.g.* 'People who drink alcohol lose control and have accidents'), and have been shown to be important determinants of an individual's decision to use substance.[13] Willner assessed alcohol expectancies as "gateway" to intake of cannabis and reported that as the frequency of drinking increased, positive cannabis expectancies increased (white circles) and negative cannabis expectancies decreased.[14] High positive expectancies of both alcohol and cannabis were associated with a low perceived self-efficacy to resist peer influence, which is considered to be a central feature in the development of problematic substance use.[9]

Personality Factors

Personality characteristics that have been linked to substance use include low assertiveness, low self-esteem, low self-confidence, low social confidence and external locus of control.[15] Psychological traits in childhood and adolescence such as alienation, impulsivity and distress can predict future drug use. Personality dimensions predictive of increased risk for substance dependence are high level of two personality characteristic; impulsivity and novelty seeking. Impulsivity appears to be a major factor in both substance dependence and borderline personality disorder. It appears more highly elevated in comorbid borderline personality disorder and substance dependence than with either disorder alone. In substance dependence subjects poor performance on gambling task suggest a heightened tendency to continue reinforce behaviour in the context of increasing negative consequences. Another trait consistently related to vulnerability to substance dependence is novelty seeking.

PSYCHOLOGICAL MANAGEMENT

Today, blending medications and psychosocial interventions in the treatment of substance abuse disorder is the norm and has considerable support in the research literature. Successful treatment of substance use disorders may involve the use of multiple specific interventions which may vary over time for any individual patient and which may involve more than one clinician. Collaborative treatment integrates medication and psychotherapy approaches for the patient.[17]

The American Psychiatric Association's Practice Guideline for Treatment of Patients with Substance Use Disorders[18] is an excellent resource on the specific psychosocial and pharmacological treatments for substance use disorders. In addition, it describes the crucial psychiatric management tasks for the psychiatrist providing integrated treatment for substance use disorders.

APA guidelines for psychiatric management of substance use disorders.

- Establishing and maintaining a therapeutic alliance
- Monitoring the patient's clinical status
- Managing intoxication and withdrawal states
- Developing and facilitating adherence to a treatment plan
- Preventing relapse, providing education about substance use disorders
- Reducing the morbidity and sequelae of substance use disorders
- Diagnosing and treating associated psychiatric disorders

PREVENTIVE MEASURES

Assessment

Before going to intervention, assessment of drug abusers is necessary in order to identify the nature and severity of the drug related problems.

Motivational Assessment

A person's level of motivation for change is an important factor in determining the likely success of any intervention,[19] gave stage of change concept. These stages can be usefully addressed in diverse problems (in addition to addictions) where change of behaviour and attitude are involved. For the field of drug and alcohol abuse, these have been adapted as follows.

Pre-Contemplation: A client is said to be in this stage when he believes that advantages from substance use outweigh its disadvantages and consequently he is not intending change in his drug using behaviour in foreseeable future.

Contemplation: This is the stage in which the client has started considering pros and cons of continuing substance use versus discontinuing or reducing it. Ambivalence is the hallmark of this stage and it is believed that pros and cons almost equal each other. The patient intends a change in the next 6 months. The therapist's role in this stage is of paramount importance and consists of tilting the balance towards the side of early change of behaviour thereby taking the client into the next stage.

Determination/Preparation: A person is said to be in this stage when he has resolved his ambivalence and is ready to participate in action oriented intervention. During this stage he also makes a choice from the available options and finalizes concrete plan of action.

Action: Overt behavioral step taken constitute action stage, for example, coming to therapist for counselling sessions, completing home assignments, and maintaining moderation of drinking.

Maintenance: After the period of intensive therapy in action stage is over, some milder amount of action is continuously required to maintain the changed behaviour; otherwise there is a risk of relapse to previous maladaptive behaviour.

Either termination or relapse: Successful observance of maintenance leads to recovery when the actions/efforts can be terminated altogether. Failure of maintenance phase leads to relapse.

To help the client move from one stage to the next one till maladaptive behaviour of hazardous use of substance is given up,[20] have recommended a unique counselling style which has been frequently used in brief interventions. It is called 'Motivational Interviewing'. Its main focus is on helping clients to explore and resolve ambivalence.

Motivational Enhancement Therapy (MET)

Motivational Enhancement Therapy (MET) aims to help the patient develop a commitment and motivation to change. The therapist adopts a focused substance use on the patient's life and collaborating with the patient to develop and implement a plan to stop using substances. MET is compatible with Prochaska and DiClemente's stages-of-change model,[19] in which patients are assessed as being in the pre-contemplation, contemplation, preparation, action, or maintenance stage of change. The patients in the contemplation stage express some willingness to change their substance use within the next 2 to 6 months, whereas those in the preparation stage are willing to make changes in the next month, but not immediately. Patients in the action stage are willing to try making changes at once, and patients in the maintenance stage have changed their behaviours consistently for atleast 3 months. However, these time frames should be viewed only as general guidelines for determining a patient's stage of change. Other factors to take into account are nonverbal behaviours and the weighs the patient gives to the pros and cons of substance use.

This model emphasizes the importance of tailoring interventions to the patient's motivational level. Interventions aimed at immediate cessation of substance use are often ineffective for patients in the contemplation and pre-contemplation stages. Unless, there is a powerful external motivator to maintain compliance (legal, employment, or family). Without an external motivator, a confrontational approach is likely to provoke resistance and treatment dropout. A realistic goal for the poorly motivated patient is to simply increase awareness of the impact of the substance use and the possibility of change. Later interventions may involve creating a change plan and discussing feelings of ambivalence, including the patient's perception of the benefits of using substances and of the reasons to stop using substances.[21]

Cue Exposure

At times environmental stimuli associated with drug taking may contribute to the continuation of drug taking behaviour. Exposure to these stimuli or cues, which cannot always be avoided in everyday life, may lead to a variety of physiological (increased heart rate, decreased skin temperature, other signs of autonomic activation) and subjective responses long after a drug user has become abstinent and usually cause craving for the drugs, diminish both the physiological and subjective responses to them.

Relapse Prevention

These methods involve the identification of high-risk situation, when there is an increased likelihood of drug taking behaviour. These may be caused by negative emotional status, interpersonal conflict or direct/indirect social pressures, and the patient is encouraged to record their use of drugs, identifying the factors that may have triggered relapse.

With help of the therapist they can analyze these situation and develop ways of dealing with them in future - perhaps by purposefully avoiding or preventing high risk situation by using structured problem solving techniques together with role playing.

Some approaches advocate graded exposure to behavioural cues; other utilizes rapid exposure (flooding). On those occasion when craving to take drug develops, techniques such as 'urge surfing are advocated allowing craving full rein, in the knowledge that it will, eventually subside. An important aspect of relapse prevention may be the distinction between lapse and relapse and how to control before relapse.

Relapse prevention is a cognitive-behavioural therapy based on the theory that the maladaptive behavioural patterns of addiction are learned and that the patient can learn to identify and correct these problematic behaviors. The therapist helps the patient achieve and maintain abstinence by helping them to better understand substance use behaviour which triggers and to improve coping skills and self-efficacy. For example, therapists teach coping and drug refusal skills to handle the stress of people, places, things, and mood states that are known to trigger relapses.[22]

CONCLUSION

There are multiple factors associated with substance abuse disorders. Such treatments may be meted out in professionally guided brief or extended interventions, or in the self-help approaches. All these, taken together, can be instrumental in achieving maintenance of abstinence, return of the drug user to the mainstream of life, and promotion of well being in the patient and his family. However, it needs to be kept in mind that pharmacological and psychosocial approaches to the management of alcohol/drug abuse tend to go hand in hand *i.e.* they are complementary to each other, and the best results have generally been obtained by a combined approach. Hence, in the treatment of patients with alcohol/drug abuse (or dependence), psychosocial management of the patient (and related family) is of equal, if not less, importance as pharmacological management.

REFERENCES

1. Caspi, D. Begg,N. Dickson, *et.al.* Personality differences predict health-risk behaviors in young adulthood: evidence from a longitudinal study. *Journal of Personality and Social Psychology*, 1997, 73, 1052-1063.
2. A.E. Skodol, J.M. Oldham, P.E. Gallaher. Axis II comorbidity of substance use disorders among patients referred for treatment of personality disorders. *American Journal Psychiatry*, 1999, 156, 733-738.
3. Edwards, G. & Gross, M.M. (1976) Alcohol dependence: Provisional description of the clinical syndrome. *British Medical Journal*, 1, 1058–1061.
4. Chen, K., & Kandel, D. B. (1995). The natural history of drug use from adolescence to the mid-thirties in a general population sample. *American journal of public health*, 85(1), 41-47.
5. Raveis, V. H., & Kandel, D. B. (1987). Changes in drug behavior from the middle to the late twenties: initiation, persistence, and cessation of use. *American Journal of Public Health,* 77(5), 607-611.
6. Horvath, A. T., Mishra, K., Epner, A. K., Cooper, G. M., (2016). Cognitive (Expectancy) Theory of Addiction and Recovery Implications. (edt by Zupanick, C. E.).
7. Gardner, M. A., (2015). Social Learning Theory: Skills Are Essential in Treating Addictive Behaviour.
8. Brown, B. B., Lohr, M. J., & McClenahan, E. L. (1986). Early adolescents' perceptions of peer pressure. *The Journal of Early Adolescence,* 6(2), 139-154.
9. Brown, B.B., Rae Clasen, D., & Eicher, S. (1986). Perceptions of peer pressure, peer conformity dispositions, and self-reported behavior among adolescents. *Developmental psychology*, 22(4), 521-530

10. Donovan, J. E., & Jessor, R. (1978). Adolescent problem drinking. Psychosocial correlates in a national sample study. *Journal of Studies on Alcohol,* 39(9), 1506-1524.

11. Jessor, R. (1987). Problem behavior theory, psychosocial development, and adolescent problem drinking. *Addiction*, 82(4), 331-342.

12. Sutherland, I., & Shepherd, J. P. (2001). Social dimensions of adolescent substance use. *Addiction*, 96(3), 445-458.

13. Brown, S. A., Goldman, M. S., & Christiansen, B. A. (1985). Do alcohol expectancies mediate drinking patterns of adults?.*Journal of Consulting and Clinical Psychology*, 53(4), 512.

14. Willner, I. R., Waters, B., Patil, S. R., Reuben, A., Morelli, J., &Riely, C. A. (2001). Ninety patients with nonalcoholic steatohepatitis: insulin resistance, familial tendency, and severity of disease. *The American journal of gastroenterology,* 96(10), 2957-2961.

15. Braucht, G. N., Brakarsh, D., Follingstad, D., & Berry, K. L. (1973). Deviant drug use in adolescence: a review of psychosocial correlates. *Psychological bulletin*, 79(2), 92.

16. American Psychiatric Association. (2000). *Diagnostic criteria from DSM-IV-TR.* American Psychiatric Pub.

17. Riba, M.B., Balon R. (1999). Psychopharmacology and Psychotherapy: A collaborative approach. Washington DC, American Psychiatric Press.

18. American Psychiatric Association (1995): Practice Guideline for Treatment of Patients with Substance Use Disorders: Alcohol, Cocaine, Opioids, Washington, DC, American Psychiatric Association.

19. Prochaska, J.O., &DiClemente, C.C. (1992). Stages of change in the modification of problem behaviours. In M. Hersen, R.M. Eisler, & P.M. Miller (Eds.), Progress in Behaviour Modification (pp. 184-214). Sycamore, IL: Sycamore Press.

20. Miller, W.R., Rollnick S. (1991).Motivational interviewing: preparing people to change addictive behaviour. New York, Guildford.

21. Miller, W.R., Zweben A, DiClemente CC, *et.al.* (1995). Motivational enhancement therapy manual. Rockville, MD: U.S. Department of Health and Human Services, National Institute of Health Publication No. 94-3723.

22. Marlatt GA, Gordon JR, (1985). Relapse Prevention: Maintenance strategies in the treatment of addictive behaviours. New York, Guilford.

Editors' Note

The management of alcohol and drug abuse go hand in hand with pharmacological and psychosocial approaches of the treatment. In the treatment of alcoholic person, the pharmacological (drug supplements) and psychological (self-determination and family support) support remain complementary to each other, and the best results have generally been obtained by a combined approach involving both approaches.

❑❑❑

10

Prohibition in India: A Study of the Historical & Contemporary Aspects

Tanushree*

Abstract

Alcoholism Prohibition has been introduced in India as well as foreign countries with the objective of reducing incidents of domestic violence, road accidents, and crimes etc. The results of such a prohibition, has been contrary to expectations as in many cases it lead to illegal sale, purchase and consumption of alcohol, and also to death of large number of people due to consumption of spurious liquor. Since, alcohol addiction is a world-wide concern hence many national and international organizations have been actively engaged in spreading awareness against its use. In India, since independence, many attempts have been made to tackle rising alcoholism. Along with treatment programs, awareness campaigns, providing medical care and counselling combined efforts of the government, NGO's and responsible citizens can prove to be of immense value in dealing with the situation.

Keywords: Alcohol, De-addiction, Prohibition, Rehabilitation

* Department of History & Civilization, Gautam Buddha University, Noida. India.

INTRODUCTION

In India, many states like Haryana, Andhra Pradesh, Tamil Nadu, Gujarat, Manipur, and Mizoram have experimented with alcohol prohibition but with limited results. Not only India, prohibition was also applied in other countries as well because of the alarming proportion of addicted individuals. From 1920-1933 the American Government introduced prohibition in order to reduce crime, improve health and avoid social problems.[1] But the results proved contrary to the expectations.[1] According to Global Status Report on Alcohol and Health, 2014 released by WHO "Up until 2025, alcohol per capita consumption is expected to continue to increase in half of the WHO regions unless effective policy responses reverse this trend. If this expected increase is not counterbalanced by substantial decrease in the other half of the WHO regions, alcohol per capita consumption globally is expected to increase"[2] The Times of India, reporting the results of a report by Paris based Organization for Economic Co-operation and Development regarding use of alcohol and its implications mentions "Among a list of 40 nations, India got the third position, only after Russian Federation and Estonia, for shooting alcohol intake between 1992-2012. Countries that closely followed were China, Israel and Brazil."[3] Thus, alcoholism is a global menace. According to National Health Portal "Alcohol use is not only restricted to men but also women. The recent trends has shown that population of women who are consuming alcohol has increased tremendously. Women are more vulnerable than men to alcohol's effects, even after drinking smaller amounts. Women who drink heavily are at a major risk of various diseases, like, osteoporosis, premature menopause, infertility and miscarriages, high blood pressure and heart disease."[4] Not even adults, even children in India are also found to be addicted to alcoholism and drugs. A study conducted by National Drug Dependence Treatment Centre (NDDTC) and AIIMS on 'Assessment of Pattern, Profile and Correlates of Substance Use among Children in India' for National Commission for Protection of Child Rights showed that "Among the total sample (n=4,024), tobacco followed by alcohol were two most common substances used over lifetime, past year or past month."[5] The report further mentions that "The current (past month) use of tobacco was reported by 79.4%, alcohol by 56.8%, inhalants by 30.5%, and cannabis by 28.9% of the sample."[5] Thus, alcoholism is growing and effecting every generation, thereby posing serious problems for not only the addicted individual but also his family and nation as well. Alcohol is also found to be responsible for marital discords, as men under the influence of alcohol are more prone to physical aggression. Parenting also gets influenced by the alcohol addiction. According to the National Commission for Protection of Child Rights study (above mentioned) the family factors that were associated with substance abuse among children were (1) Substance use in a family member (57%); (2) Single parent/ broken families/living with relatives/ no parents (25%); (3) Fights in the family (46.6%); and (4) History of physical/ verbal abuse (45.3%).[5] This proves that children in whose family, a member was addicted to substance abuse, that child was more prone to substance abuse. The entire family gets affected by addicted individual as socially, the family gets stigmatized or even secluded. Relationships within the family too are not healthy, due to neglecting of duties by the alcoholic person and even relations at the workplace are affected. An addicted person is not able to contribute fully towards his official duties because of his drinking habits; this might lead to him losing his job, reputation and social respect.

A few Indian states has reacted to this menace by implementing prohibition expecting to lower down incidents of accidents, crime, domestic violence. According to Deccan Chronicle, "India is among the leading countries when it comes to deaths due to road accidents. Around 410 people die every day in road traffic accidents in India. Around 1.5 lakh lives were lost in 2016 due to road accidents, and drunk driving was responsible for 40-50% of the accidents."[6] Alcoholism also leads to economic loss for the family. According to Global Status Report on Alcohol, 2004 by WHO "In India household expenditure on alcohol varies between 3% to 45% of income. Alcohol abuse is one of the main killers of young men in India today. However, its real impact is on the social and family dynamics that underlie its communities."[7] Apart from the above mentioned harmful consequences of alcohol consumption, it also has serious implications for the health of the addicted individual. It may lead to neuropsychiatric disorder, cardiovascular diseases, Cirrhosis of Liver etc. depending on the age, sex and pattern of alcohol consumption. Alcohol addiction as a serious global issue and in recent times it has received international attention. World Health Organization on 21st May, 2010, in the Sixty-third session of World Health Assembly adopted a resolution WHA63.13, endorsing a 'Global Strategy to Reduce Harmful Use of Alcohol'.[8] According to the Strategy, the four priority areas for global action were as follows;[8]

Public health advocacy and partnership;
Technical support and capacity building;
Production and dissemination of knowledge;
Resource Mobilization

Historical Background: After independence in 1947, states like Gujarat introduced prohibition. According to an article published in India Today on 30th September, 1977 "With the advent of Independence, a number of states, largely under the influence of Mahatma Gandhi, introduced an active prohibition policy. Bombay achieved total prohibition in 1951 by progressively increasing the number of weekly dry days. Gujarat adopted the Bombay Prohibition Act when the state came into being in 1960. Mysore (now Karnataka), Orissa, Assam, Madhya Pradesh, Punjab and Delhi went partially dry, while Bihar, Jammu & Kashmir, Rajasthan, U.P. and West Bengal opted to stay wet. The period saw an alarming drop in excise revenue and an equally alarming spurt in the distillation of bootleg liquor."[9]Public opinion, especially of women citizens has always been in favor of alcohol prohibition, and at many places citizens themselves participated or initiated movements against addiction. According to Fahey, Blocker & Tyrell (2003) "Andhra Pradesh and other states witnessed grassroots movements against *arrack*, popular local liquor among peasants that was charged with causing domestic violence and impoverishing families. Also Tamil Nadu introduced prohibition measures, of which vestiges still survive at the end of twentieth century."[10] In 1954, the Planning Commission, of Government of India had set up a Prohibition Enquiry Committee in order to make recommendations on this issue. Another Committee named Tek Chand Committee was appointed in 1964 by Government of India in order to look into the prohibition issue. Many committees were appointed after independence, for instance Prohibition Enquiry Committee (1954), Central Prohibition Committee (1960), Study Team Prohibition (1963), Expert Committee (1972) and Drug Addiction Committee (1976).[11] In the year 1986, a non-profit organization named Alcoholics Anonymous (AA) was reportedly very successful in alcohol de-addiction. According to India Today, "AA is a non-profit world-wide organization of recovered alcoholics trying to help others in the same plight. There are already 100 such groups in the country, with Bombay (now Mumbai) alone boasting 55. Other cities with AA groups are Bangalore, Goa, Madras (now Chennai), Secunderabad, New Delhi, Cochin, Mangalore, Nagpur, Pune and Mysore."[12]

Recent Cases: Some of such recent examples includes when in order to fulfill a poll promise Chief Minister of Haryana Shri Bansi Lal, ordered ban on manufacture, sale and consumption of alcohol in Haryana in 1996 but enforcement of such a ban proved to be very difficult. According to a report published in India Today "The official count as of mid-August reads 3,561 persons arrested since prohibition was enforced on July 1, 3278 cases registered, 28,528 bottles and 13,720 pouches seized, 70 illicit distilleries destroyed. In some police stations, there is no place left for seized stocks."[13] However, the ban was lifted from 1st April, 1998 onwards due to "large scale smuggling and liquor mafia."[14] Haryana government also notified a scheme for giving awards for "Outstanding services rendered by individuals and institutions in the prevention of abuse of alcohol, narcotic drugs, psychotropic substances and other addictive substances like cough syrups and correction fluid."[15] Awards are given to Non-profit organization, educational institutions, municipal or Panchayat organizations and also individuals etc. for their contribution in alcohol prevention. Also in February 2017 Haryana government banned the consumption of liquor in vehicles and imposition of a fine of ₹ 5000 if caught drinking in vehicles.[16] Delhi government in 2016 had imposed a similar ban. The reason behind such steps is to prevent road accidents as well as to reduce crime. Similarly, in Bihar from 1st April, 2016 prohibition was imposed by Nitish Kumar's government.[17] The Bihar government has also set up 39 de-addiction centers and counselling centers in order to help people in de-addiction.[18] In total 3,645 people were arrested and 3,859 cases of violation of alcohol prohibition were lodged in Bihar. A total of 34,470 raids were conducted after prohibition in Bihar.[19] Recently, in December 2016 Supreme Court ordered closure of all liquor shops along national and state highways; the Haryana Government anticipating a loss of 50% revenue, sought legal assistance in order to find an alternative.[20] Consequently, in March 2017 the Supreme Court of India relaxed the distance and directed that for municipal areas having less than 20,000 population situated on highways, the distance of 500 meters was reduced to 220 meters.[21]

Such steps have received special appreciation from women who happen to suffer a lot due to addicted husbands. It has also been seen that prohibition has also resulted in deaths due to consumption of illegal alcohol. According to an article published in Hindustan Times "India has a recurring problem of poisoned or spurious liquor though it is not limited to states with prohibition. In July 2009, 136 people died in Gujarat after consuming hooch. In June 2015, 95 people died after drinking illegal liquor in Mumbai."[22] The Indian Express also reported that "Five people died everyday in 2014 after drinking spurious liquor. In 2015, consumption of illegally brewed liquor claimed that more than 100 lives in Malwani and Mumbai, triggering widespread outrage. As many as 1,699 people died in 2014 after consuming spurious/illicit liquor, an increase of 339 percent from 387 in 2013."[23] Similarly, in August 2016, 13 people died in Bihar's Gopalganj district after consumption of country made illicit liquor.[24] Thus we see that prohibition failed to achieve its objectives and had to be lifted after some time in many cases.

De-Addiction: From time to time, for the victims of alcoholism and drug abuse the Government of India, has launched many schemes to help people in de-addiction and also to increase awareness concerning rehabilitation, treatment and prevention of the individuals suffering from addiction. In 1998, a National Centre for Drug Abuse Prevention was set up by Government of India at New Delhi with the primary objective of raising the standard of professionals in de-addiction centers, updating of data & information, standardization of care and monitoring system. In July 2008, National Consultative Committee on De-addiction and Rehabilitation was formed, to help government in framing out measures to address the problem of rising alcoholism in the country. A sub-committee under the above mentioned Committee was formed in order to "draft a National Policy on Prevention of Alcoholism and Substance Abuse and Rehabilitation of Victims".[25] The Ministry of Social Justice and Empowerment also came up with a new initiative in 2014 called "National Policy for Drug Demand Reduction" to cater to the problems of alcoholism as well as misuse of medicine. Under this Policy the main purpose is to sensitize the youth about the harmful effects of alcohol. The objectives of the Government of India Scheme (effective from 1st January, 2015) for Prevention of Alcoholism and Substance (Drug) Abuse, 2015 are as follows;[26]

- To create awareness and educate people about the ill-effects of alcoholism and substance abuse on the individual, the family, the workplace and society at large;

- To provide for the whole range of community based services for the identification, motivation, counselling, de-addiction, after care and rehabilitation for Whole Person Recovery (WPR) of addicts to make a person drug free, crime free and gainfully employed;
- To alleviate the consequences of drug and alcohol dependence among the individual, the family, and society at large;
- To facilitate, research, training and documentation and collection of relevant information to strengthen the above mentioned objectives; and
- To support other activities which are in accordance with the mandate of the Ministry of Social Justice and Empowerment in this field.

However, what should be ensured is that these measures or steps should reach the lower sections of society, who suffer the most when their breadwinner gets addicted to alcohol, and as a consequence wastes meager family resources on alcohol and also suffers from medical complexities which the family is usually not in a position to deal with. Many NGO's too have been involved in helping people in de-addiction. International organizations too contributed in the fight against alcoholism and many projects with international organizations were initiated, for instance "Between 1994 and the end of 1999, the International Labour Organization implemented a project to develop community-based rehabilitation and workplace prevention programmes in India. Agreements were signed with 12 enterprises, with a combined workforce of over 110,000, and key management officials and their partners in NGOs were all provided with training."[27] According to Times Now report, an average of 20 people, mostly below 35yrs of age arrive at the state run de-addiction centre in Haryana every day.[28] This is the situation in many of the Indian states. Keeping in mind the growing number of women addicts in Punjab, the government is planning to set up an exclusive women de-addiction centre in Kapurthala District.[29]

Government has also included NGO's in many of its schemes for rehabilitation purposes. According to Scheme of Assistance for Prevention of Alcoholism and Substance (Drugs) Abuse and for Social Defense Services, 2015 almost 350-400 Integrated Rehabilitation Centres for Addicts are working with the support of Ministry of Social Justice and Empowerment.[30] Apart from it "The Ministry is also supporting Twelve NGO's working in the field of drug abuse prevention to function as

Regional Resource and Training Centres (RRTC's) for imparting training in local cultural setting to the service providers working in various IRCA's and for undertaking advocacy, research and monitoring for drug abuse programmes."[30] Awareness generation and de-addiction programmes has been the primary focus of government initiatives as the future generations should be well aware of the consequences of alcohol addiction, in order to live a healthy life.

CONCLUSION

Alcoholism today, is a global concern because of its adverse consequences not only from the physical health perspective, but also because alcohol consumption becomes an addict's priority hence he/she often neglects responsibility towards family members, indulges in violent behavior, increases financial strain on family etc. which results in considerable social and moral degradation of the person concerned. While prohibition may prove to be deterrent for some, it is not a long term solution to the problem of alcoholism. Citizen participation along with government initiatives together can go a long way in dealing with the menace of alcoholism.

REFERENCES

1. Singh, Joginder. (8 september, 2014). "The Many Problems with Prohibition", (Online Web), Accessed 24 May, 2017 URL: http://www.dailypioneer.com/columnists/edit/the-many-problems-with-prohibition.html.
2. Global Status Report on Alcohol and Health, 2014 by WHO.
3. Roy, Sumitra. (17 May 2015). "Indians drinking alcohol up 55% in 20 years", (Online Web), Accessed 26 May, 2017 URL: http://timesofindia.indiatimes.com/india/Indians-drinking-alcohol-up-55-in-20-years/articleshow/47313965.cms
4. National Health Portal. "Quit Alcoholism", (Online Web), Accessed 29 May, 2017 URL: https://www.nhp.gov.in/quit-alcoholism_pg
5. National Commission for Protection of Child Rights. Report on 'Assessment of Pattern, Profile and Correlates of Substance Use Among Children In India' 2013.
6. Matcheswala, Y.A. (14 May, 2017). "Road Menace: Drugs in Race with Drinks on the Highway", (Online Web), Accessed 26 May, 2017 URL: dhttp://www.deccanchronicle.com/nation/current-affairs/140517/road-menace-drugs-in-race-with-drinks-on-the-highway.html

7. WHO. Global Status Report on Alcohol, 2004. (Online Web), Accessed 29 May, 2017 URL: http://www.who.int/substance_abuse/publications/en/india.pdf

8. WHO. Global Strategy to reduce harmful use of alcohol. Online Web), Accessed 29 May, 2017 URL: http://www.who.int/substance_abuse/activities/gsrhua/en/

9. Bobb, Dilip. (30 September, 1977).”Prohibition: Going dry with Desai”, (Online Web), Accessed 25 May, 2017 URL: http://indiatoday.intoday.in/story/pm-morarji-desai-determined-to-enforce-total-prohibition-on-liquor-consumption/1/435846.html

10. J.S. Blocker, D.M. Fahey, I.R. Tyrrell. Alcohol and Temperance in Modern History: An International Encyclopedia., Vol 1, ABC-CLIO: California, **2003**.

11. P.M. Miller, T.D. Nirenberg. Prevention of Alcohol Abuse, Plenum Press: New York, **2012**.

12. Chengappa, Raj. (30 April, 1986). “De-addiction: Creditable Successes” (Online Web), Accessed 28 May 2017 URL: http://indiatoday.intoday.in/story/one-of-the-most-successful-ways-of-treating-addicts-is-alcoholics-anonymous-programme/1/348374.html

13. Parihar, Rohit (15 September, 1996). “The Other Side of Prohibition” (Online Web), Accessed 29 May, 2017 URL: indiatoday.intoday.in/story/ban-on-alcohol-proves-to-be-mixed-blessing in Haryana/1/283131.html.

14. Gaur, Sanjeev (18 March, 1998). “Haryana to lift Prohibition from April 1”, (Online Web), Accessed 1 June, 2017 URL: www.business-standard.com/article/specials/haryana-to-lift-prohibition-from-April1-19803180160_1.html.

15. Many schemes have been initiated in order to encourage people to stop the use of alcohol.

16. TNN (15 February, 2017). “Haryana to fine people ₹ 5,000 for drinking in a car”, (Online Web), Accessed 28 May, 2017 URL: www.timesofindia.indiatimes.com/city/gurgaon/haryana-to-fine-people-rs-5000-for-drinking-in-car-/articlesshow/57155517.cms.

17. This was a result of a poll promise which was highly supported by women in the state.

18. IANS (20 September, 2016). “After Liquor Ban, Bihar Government to Focus on De-addiction”, (Online Web), Accessed 29 May, 2017 URL: http://www.thehindu.com/news/national/other-states/After-liquor-ban-Bihar-government-to-focus-on-de-addiction/article14216353.ece

19. PTI. (1 June, 2016). "Over 91,000 liters of liquor seized in Bihar in past two months, 3,645 arrested", (Online Web), Accessed 29 May, 2017 http://indianexpress.com/article/india/india-news-india/over-91000-litres-of-liquor-seized-in-bihar-in-past-2-months-3645-arrested-2829389/

20. Siwach, Sukhbir. (26 January, 2017). "Haryana: Liquor ban on Highways could cost state Rs 2,500 crore", (Online Web), Accessed 3 June, 2017 URL:www.indianexpress.com/article/india/haryana-Liquor-ban-on-highways-could-cost- state-rs- 2,500-crore-4492019

21. Praksh, Satya. (31 March, 2017). "Supreme Court cuts highway liquor ban distance from 500 m to 220 m in small towns", (Online Web), Accessed 30 May, 2017 URL: http://www.tribuneindia.com/news/nation/supreme-court-cuts-highway-liquor-ban-distance-from-500m-to-220m-in-small-towns/385114.html

22. Siddiqui, F.A. (17 April, 2016). "A chequered history: Does Alcohol prohibitionreallyworkinIndia",(OnlineWeb),Accessed29May,2017URL: http://www.hindustantimes.com/india/a-chequered-history-does-alcohol-prohibition-really-work-in-india/story-dR7CYZVLDvzLdkDe9wKo1H.html

23. IANS (25 May, 2016). "One Indian Dies every 96 minutes due to alcohol consumption", (Online Web), Accessed 26 May, 2017 URL: http://indianexpress.com/article/lifestyle/life-style/one-indian-dies-every-96-minutes-due-to-alcohol-consumption-2818493/

24. Azad, Nayear. (18 August, 2016). "Hooch tragedy in Bihar claims 13", (Online Web), Accessed 29 May, 2017 URL:http://www.asianage.com/india/hooch-tragedy-dry-bihar-claims-13-931

25. Sharma, Neetu. (1 December, 2014). "Government mulls strategy to save youth from alcoholism and Pharmaceutical drug abuse", (Online Web), Accessed 30 May, 2017 URL: http://indiatoday.intoday.in/story/drug-abuse-alcoholism-cannabis-opium-heroin-government-npddr-ministry-of-social-justice-and-empowerment/1/404530.html

26. Scheme of Assistance for Prevention of Alcoholism and Substance (Drugs) Abuse and for Social Defence Services, 2015, Ministry o Social Justice and Empowerment, GOI.

27. ILO (2003). Alcohol and Drug Problems at Work: The Shift to Prevention. International Labour Organization, Geneva.

28. TNN (4 July 2016). (Online Web), Accessed 30 May, 2017 URL: http://www.timesnow.tv/india/video/haryana-government-rehabs-get-about-20-youths-daily-even-14-year-olds-on-a-high/45384.

29. Akzher, Adil. (11 May, 2017). "Punjab to get first government run de-addiction centre for women only", (Online Web), Accessed 2 June, 2017 URL: http://indianexpress.com/article/india/punjab-to-get-first-govt-run-de-addiction-centre-for-women-only-4650496/

30. Scheme of Assistance for Prevention of Alcoholism and Substance (Drugs) Abuse and for Social Defence Services, 2015.

Editors' Note

The proposition of prohibition (by state litigations) in recent past and contemporary time as well may prove to be deterrent. The complete prohibition is not a long term solution to the problem of alcoholism due to ill social issues that arise due to impact of it. Citizen participation along with government initiatives together can go a long way in dealing with the menace of alcoholism. Awareness about adverse effect has proved a tool of choice to combat the wide spread alcoholism.

❑❑❑

11

Patterns of Alcohol Abuse Among Urban Slums & Substandard Settlements: Review of Indian Literature Towards Implications for Policy Interventions

Sushil Kumar* and Gurpreet Kaur**

Abstract

Alcoholism has emerged as one of the gravest public health concern worldwide. In India, despite ban on alcohol in many states like Gujarat, Manipur, Bihar etc. millions of families are getting affected by alcoholism. Due to its growing menace of ill effects, many social activists, medical professionals, law makers, and public are making efforts for necessary intervention programs. Today, in spite of many awareness programs, there is a gross absence of information on the extent of prevalence and various patterns of alcohol consumption in India. The present chapter highlights the key findings of various research studies related to alcohol abuse among residents of urban slums and substandard settlements. It also summaries the observations of

* Department of Social Work, Jamia Millia Islamia, New Delhi.

** Defence Institute of Psychological Research, DRDO, New Delhi.

the interactions made during field visits to different slums in Delhi and National Capital Region.

Keywords: alcoholism pattern, slum, policy.

INTRODUCTION

Alcohol abuse is a major public health problem. It is a causal factor in more than 60 major types of diseases; these majorly include several types of cancer, hemorrhagic stroke and hypertensive heart disease, cardiovascular diseases, liver cirrhosis and neuropsychiatric diseases. According to Organization for Economic Cooperation and Development (OECD), during 1992-2012, the per capita consumption of alcohol in India has increased by whopping 55%, the third highest increase in the world, after Russian Federation and Estonia. An epidemiological survey[1] was conducted by the department of psychiatry, Govt. Medical College and Hospital, Chandigarh to estimate the pattern of alcohol and other substance dependence in rural and slum dwellers population of Chandigarh. It was observed that 6.88% individuals of the total population surveyed (2992) fulfilled the dependence criteria of ICD-10. The study found that alcohol is the main element of dependence for large number of urban slum dwellers who indulge into substance abuse and rural areas abusers. Age at first drug use was 20.89 5.31 years (mean ± S.D) among rural population and 19.75 ± 5.4 years (mean ± SD) in urban slums. The study pointed that people starts alcohol and become dependent even before their legal age of purchasing alcohol . Majority of them reported having health related complications (85.71%) followed by family problems (77.31%) due to drug dependence. The results of the study also indicate towards alcohol abuse as the major factor for family disputes and poor health. This survey reflects the need to intensify efforts at the community level to reach the unreached.[1]

Das *et.al.* (2006) studied the health and social impact of alcohol in India. The study submitted that different cultures have varied impact on the pattern of alcohol consumption.[4] Therefore, it is necessary to evolve specific and customized policies that target the reduction of impact of alcoholism in our societies. The intervention needs to address issues at both ends that is market of alcohol related beverages and alcohol abuse by the society. It is a matter of debate whether government should allow access to alcohol beverages and soldering their responsibilities by simply arguing that warning has been placed on all alcohol related beverages.

In one of the study supported by Regional Office for South-East Asia (WHO SEARO) conducted by the National Institute of Mental Health and Neurosciences (NIMHANS) assessed the problem of alcohol and its impact on socio-economic factors in a sampled population.[16] Information was collected from 3258 respondents of age ranging between 16 and 60 years. The samples were drawn from varied locations including urban, rural, town, and slum areas. The study focused to assess both the qualitative and quantitative factors that had an impact on alcohol abuse. The study reveals that alcohol impacts drastically both the abusers and their family constituents. It also highlighted that approximately 33% respondents indulge into alcohol abuse regularly on the pretext of self-styled reasoning and approximately 2% of women respondents consume alcohol on a regular basis.

Ghose *et.al.*, (2009) conducted a cross-sectional community-based study to examine the forms of alcohol abuse by male adults in a slum in West Bengal, India.[6] Post literature review, an interview schedule was designed on consultation with experts of public health. The study utilized Alcohol-Use Disorders Identification Test (AUDIT) questionnaire – a tool for screening the excessive drinking. Moreover, the tool of data collection has had variables focusing on the age of drinking alcohol, period of pattern of current drinking, nature of alcoholic beverages, drinking network of people, the time of drinking alcohol, favorite place of drinking, nature of source of alcohol beverages, views on drinking and concerns. The study reveals that slum inhabitants are the main victims of alcohol abuse because of their abysmal socio-economic situation. It impacts the slum dwellers in their physical, mental, social and cultural domains. The study revealed that the prevalence of current alcohol consumers was 66%. On AUDIT score, 78% of current alcohol consumers had a non-hazardous and non-harmful pattern, 8% of the people exhibited a hazardous alcohol usage and 14% showed complete dependence on alcohol. The mean age of the consumers was 31.4±10.8 years. Amongst the alcohol-dependents, approximately 50% aged 50-59 years whereas 17.6% aged 30-39 years. The most productive age of 20-39 had all the hazardous or harmful respondents. The results also points that large part of the income is spent on the alcohol than meeting the family needs. The study found that mean age was more (38.7±13.9) of the alcohol-dependents was as compared to non-hazardous non-harmful and hazardous or harmful consumers (30.5±10.8 and 28.8±5.7 respectively).

The mean age 20.5±5.7 years was recoded as the age of initiation of alcohol use among the respondents. This study also supports the early age drinking habit among the slum dwellers. It suggests that there are greater number of chances that majority of current drinkers actually start drinking before the legal age of drinking. The study found that mean duration of alcohol drinking is 6.7±5.8 years.

In a cross sectional study, Goswami (2010) examined the socio-demographic and environmental profiles as well as magnitude of morbidity among urban slum dwellers.[9] The literacy rate was 16.8 % and 5.6% among males and females respondents respectively. Among five years above age males, 27%, 9.7% and 7.4% had a habit of smoking, tobacco chewing and alcohol intake respectively. Among five years above age females 4.36 %, 10.9% and 0.84 % had a habit of smoking, tobacco chewing and alcohol intake respectively.

Alcohol is counted as one of the leading factor for death and disability in India. Statistics on volume and nature of consumption are crucial to shape policies and intervention programs. Girish *et.al.*, (2010) conducted a study to enlist the spectrum and form of alcohol abuse in different communities residing in rural, urban, town and sub-settlements.[8] A household survey was conducted using simple random sampling methodology. Overall, 13% of males and females consumed alcohol. Proportion of users was greater in town (15.7%) and among 26-45 years (67.4%). The study indicates that most productive age is major section of people who indulge into substance abuse. This alcoholism poses a greater risk of poor marital relationships, risk of serious health problems, and continuing to have poor socio-economic status. Whisky (49%) and arrack (35%) were the most favored alcohol beverages. The rural respondents preferred the arrack whereas urban respondents preferred beer. Around 70% respondents were long-term alcohol abuser and the magnitude was higher in rural and town locations. The study recorded 17% respondents as heavy-users. The regular and frequent excess drinkers were respondents from rural and slum areas. Beside residential status, peer pressure was recorded as the core factor for indulging into alcohol abuse. Majority of the respondents preferred liquor-shops, bars, pubs, and restaurants as place of drinking.

In a community based cross-sectional door to door field survey, the Prakash *et al* (2010) examined the role played by socio-demographic factors in perpetuating the habit of drug abuse.[5] The study had respondents of both sex who had age of 15 and above. The study used the two staged systematic sampling to draw samples from households and examine the drug abuse and correlations with socio-demographic variables. Through a structured interview schedule samples were drawn from urban slum community in Mumbai, India. The study observed that approximately 50% of respondents were found to be positive for drug abuse of single or multiform of drug. Approximately 60% drug abusers fall in the age range of 15 to 34 years (academic and career building age). This study also indicates towards early age drinking habits among the habitants of poor substandard settlements. 65.2% males reported to having their first use of any drug while in the age range of 15-24 years 72.1% of drug abusers were recorded to be either illiterate or below middle pass. It shows that drug peddlers target the people in their early ages. The study highlights that people in young age, with illiteracy, poor working status & low socio-demographic factors are prone to drug abuse. It also indicated towards role of peer pressure while initiating abuse of any drug.

Domestic violence is the major threat to women's health and development in India. It is regarded that alcohol is core factor for domestic violence for women slum dwellers. In a Kolkata based study on slum women Sinha *et.al.* (2012) examined the domestic violence faced by married women.[15] It was observed that alcohol addiction in the family is an important contributor towards domestic violence in slum families. Majority of the study show a direct correlation between alcohol abuse and family problems including marital disputes.

In another study, Kumar *et.al.* (2013) examined the magnitude and nature of alcohol use by utilizing Alcohol Use Disorders Identification Test (AUDIT) in rural parts of Tamil Nadu.[11] For this community based cross sectional research, 946 respondents of age 10 and above were interviewed. Data on alcohol abuse was collected by utilizing 'Alcohol Use Disorder Identification Test' (AUDIT) tool. Data on nature and correlated factors like socio-demographic details, habit of smoking, habit of tobacco chewing and prevalence of chronic diseases were collected through a well formed structured questionnaire. Study found prevalence of alcohol use to be 9.4%. Prevalence was more among male respondents 16.8%) as compared to female respondents (1.3%). Mean age of alcohol abuse initiation was recorded to be 25.3 +9.0 years, a most productive age of the people.

Mohanan (2013) attempts to record the magnitude of alcohol abuse, tobacco abuse and sexual behaviour among younger people living in urban localities in Udupi region of Karnataka state.[12] The aim of study was to assess the relationship between drug abuse and risky sexual behaviour among adolescents. It also aimed to draw linkages between potentially socio-economic factors impacting the sexual behavior of adolescents in inebriated situations. A sample of 376 adolescents (in the age range of 15-19 years) studying in different schools and colleges was collected. The study utilized the Youth Risk Behavior Survey questionnaire and guidelines for drawing data from the population. Respondents' alcohol consumption pattern, habits of smoking and risky sexual behaviour patterns were examined. The magnitude of alcohol abuse, tobacco intake and risky sexual activity was recorded to occur in 5.7%, 7.2% and 5.5% of respondents respectively. The mean age of the respondents' first sexual experience, intake of alcohol and tobacco use was reported to be around 16.8 years. This indicates towards need of a comprehensive intervention on sexual health of adolescents in the country. The religion and existence of tobacco user in the family were important factors. The prevalence of multiple risk behaviours clearly indicate towards an integrated and multi-disciplinary approach of intervention. Health education at various stages be it family, community, school be utilized to enhance the knowledge and information of parents and adolescents.

Raj *et.al.* (2013) conducted a study on alcoholism among youth. It was intended to analyze the socio economic conditions and problem among alcoholics in Tamil Nadu.[13] The respondents were selected from five slums of Trichy. The study found that most of respondents were literate and people were spending around two to four thousand per month on their alcohol. Such large proportion of earning when spent on alcohol, there are much greater chances that children and women would be denied for many needs. This will cause a serious family dispute and day-to-day violence. It was found that 92% of the total respondents had their first drinks with their friends. Majority (70%) of the respondents started their first drink for the purpose of pleasure. This study found that respondents spent minimum of Rs.100 for a drink when they go for it. Most of them (60%) felt that their habit of alcohol intake neither brings down the family status nor it downs their own individual status. 70% respondents were well aware about the ill-effects of alcohol intake through various sources but more than 90% of respondents were not willing to be away from habit of alcohol intake.

Ghulam *et.al.* (2016) attempted to understand the prevalence and nature of drug abuse in slum inhabitants.[7] For the study Prakash Chandra Sethi Nagar' slum area located in Indore district of Madhya Pradesh was targeted. At the outset, an awareness camp on drug abuse was conducted with the leaders, key persons, and local community people. Post camp, door to door household survey was conducted. The information was collected from respondents comprising of all the family members. The study recorded the prevalence rate of 56% populations. There were 78.2% males, and 28.2% females. It was also observed that 72% of the respondents who were drug abusers had been working as laborers. It is very evident in most studies that a significant number of women also indulge into alcoholism in slums and substandard settlements. This calls for serious consideration by policy makers to deal with drug and alcoholism in slums.

Begum *et.al.* (2015), conducted across-sectional community based household survey in two urban slums of Mumbai in Maharashtra to examine the socio-demographic factors associated with domestic violence.[3] The women who had atleast one child were chosen for the study through cluster systematic random sampling. The study collected the data on socio-demographic variables, reproductive and domestic violence history through a face to face interview method. The study recorded that the prevalence of female residing in slum experience domestic violence was 21.2%. It was also found that instances of domestic violence were higher in cases of husband being alcoholic (RR: 2.17, (95% CI: 1.58-2.98). The findings show that the increased risk of domestic violence was rampant in urban slums. The study found significant association between domestic violence and variables such as early marriage, working status of women, and cultural factors.

Sachdeva *et.al.* (2016) studied the alcohol consumption patterns among males in rural Haryana.[14] The study had 345 selected interviews using semi-structured interview schedule. The finding shows that mean age of the sampled adult male was 46.6 (±14.2) years. Around 64.6% had only 5 years of education, 46.4% were recorded to be farmers, 54.2% respondents lived in joint family system and 59.7% recorded their monthly family income as upto Rs. 10,000. Around 43% of the respondents were well aware about ill and adverse impact of alcohol abuse. Around 94% respondents of the study had consumed alcohol atleast once. Around 66% respondents had consumed country liquor. 73.3% of the respondents took alcohol either at their own house or at their friend's house. The study found that 86.2% of the respondents purchased alcohol from village shop and on an average people spent Rs. 500 to 900 per month on their liquor intake habit. 38% of the respondents had no eatables while consuming alcohol. Out of the total respondents, around 60% were recorded as alcohol dependent and around 40% recognized it as a problem and wanted to get rid from it. Such studies indicate a close proximity between rural areas and slums on the alcoholism.

IMPLICATIONS FOR POLICY INTERVENTION

In India, alcoholism is turning to be a growing public health concern. There is widespread agreement that human capital loss from alcohol will grow even larger, unless effective interventions and policies are implemented to curb the alcohol menace in the country. In an alarming revelation, the Global Status report on alcohol and health 2014, released by the World Health Organization (WHO) states that the amount of alcohol consumption has raised in India between the periods of 2008 to 2012. 11% of the population in India indulged in heavy or binge-drinking. In India, drinking age varies from state to state ranging from 18 to 27 years. But, modernization, urbanization, and globalization have impacted the adolescents and more and more children are becoming regular alcohol abusers. The minors residing in slums and sub settlements indulging into regular drinking habits has become a major concern for development experts and social scientists.

CONCLUSION

The present chapter is an attempt to review various studies related to alcohol abuse in different parts of the country, India and its correlates. As observed, alcohol abuse is directly linked to poor socio-economic status of families in slum or substandard settlements, thus there is strong need that policies and programmes must cater to socio-economic needs of the people. There is urgent need that policy makers create adequate space for effective intervention to combat the menace of alcohol abuse in the country. The Constitution of India states, 'The State shall endeavor to bring about prohibition of the consumption of intoxicating drinks.' The Alcohol Abuse Information & Resource Centre (AAIC) must be opened in slum areas and substandard settlements to focus on Behaviour Change Communication (BCC) activities. The scaling up of Alcoholics Anonymous in all major districts will benefit the alcoholics to live a better life. Health educational interventions among those who are at a higher risk and management of alcohol dependent subjects should be addressed simultaneously.

REFERENCES

1. B.S. Chavan, P. Arun, R. Bhargava, G.P. Singh. Prevalence of alcohol and drug dependence in rural and slum population of Chandigarh: A community survey. *IJP* **2007**, 49(1), 44–48.
2. T. Bardhan, A.M. Saikia, R. Baruah. Substance use among adolescents living in slums of Guwahati city, Assam: A growing public health concern. *Int J Med PH* **2015**, 5, 279-82.
3. S. Begum, B. Donta, S. Nair, C.P. Prakasam. Socio-demographic factors associated with domestic violence in urban slums, Mumbai, Maharashtra, India. *IJMR*, **2015**, 141(6), 783–788.
4. S.K. Das, V. Balakrishnan, D.M. Vasudevan. Alcohol: its health and social impact in India. *NMJI*, **2006**, 19(2), 94.
5. Din, Prakash, Ranjan,Namita, R. M. Chaturvedi. A study of socio-demographic factors contributing to the habit of drug abuse in the urban slum community of Mumbai. Biomedical Research. Allied Academies **2010**.
6. S. Ghosh, A. Samanta, S. Mukherjee. Patterns of Alcohol Consumption among Male Adults at a Slum in Kolkata, India. *JHPN* **2012**, 30(1), 73–81.
7. R. Ghulam, K. Verma, P. Sharma, M. Razdan, A. Rahul. Drug abuse in slum population. *IJP* **2016**, 58(1), 83-86.
8. N. Girish, R. Kavita, G. Gururaj, V. Benegal. Alcohol Use and Implications for Public Health: Patterns of Use in Four Communities. *IJCM* **2010**, 35(2), 238–244.
9. M. Goswami, G. Kedia. Socio-Demographic and Morbidity Profile of
10. Slum Area in Ahmedabad, India, *NJCM*, **2010**, 1(2), 106-110.
11. S. Kim, S. Rifkin, S.M. John, K.S. Jacob. Nature, prevalence and risk factors of alcohol use in an urban slum of Southern India. *NMJI*, **2013**. 26 (4), 203-209.
12. S. Kumar, Ganesh *et.al.* Prevalence and Pattern of Alcohol Consumption Using AUDIT in Rural Tamil Nadu, India. *JCDR* **2013**, 1637–1639.
13. P. Mohanan, S. Swain, N. Sanah, V. Sharma, D. Ghosh. A Study on the Prevalence of Alcohol Consumption, Tobacco Use and Sexual Behaviour among Adolescents in Urban Areas of the Udupi District, Karnataka, India. *SQUMJ* **2014**, 14(1), 104–112.

14. M. Raj, R.M. Asir, S. Tamilenthi. A study on alcoholism among youth residing in Trichirappalli slums, Tamil Nadu, India. *AJSR*, **2013**. 2(2), 01-07.
15. S. Sachdeva, M. Nagar, A.K. Tyagi, R. Sachdeva. Alcohol Consumption Practices Amongst Adult Males in a Rural Area of Haryana. Medical Journal of Dr. D.Y. Patil University **2016**. 7 (2), 01-07.
16. S. Sinha, S. Mallik, S. Sanyal, D. Dasgupta, A. Pal. Mukherjee. Domestic violence among ever married women of reproductive age group in a slum of Kolkata. *IJPH*, **2016**, 56(1), 31-6.
17. WHO. Burden and socio-economic impact of alcohol: the Bangalore study 2006. WHO Regional Office for South-East Asia, New Delhi.

Editors' Note

The literature analysis for various incidences and research studies related reports have been source of indirect inferences. It can be used as indication of relative prevalence of alcoholism in urban and slum areas. Time to time reports of alcoholism specific cases and related violence (domestic, social, peer group fights etc.) indicate higher prevalent of alcoholism in poor slum areas.

12

Alcoholism: Popular Culture and Narrative therapy Interventions

Ruby*

Abstract

The chapter is a critical reflection on the representation of alcohol consumption in popular culture. Normalization of drinking practice due to frequent positive references to alcohol in media has regressive consequences. Elitism, glamour, masculinity and power are put under one canopy in popular culture. Critical side-effects of alcoholism are rarely mentioned in mainstream visual media such as television programs and cinema. The discussion here is to make readers aware how positive portrayal of drinking is an accomplice in widening the chasm between gender binaries. Gender and identity are two intertwined concepts. Identity is subject to the narrative created by an individual about his life. Hence, Narrative therapy can be very useful to counter such misguiding practices. The theory of Simulation and Simulacra has been used to analyze deep-rooted psychological effects of alcohol consumption on its consumers.

Keywords: Popular culture, Media, Gender binaries, Alcoholism, Simulation and Simulacra, Narrative therapy

* Department of Applied Science, Maharaja Surajmal Institute of Technology, Janak Puri, New Delhi-110058. India.

INTRODUCTION

The cultures of time impact the prevalence of norms in the society and level of portrayal of norms impact the promotion or cessation of acceptable behavior in society.

The chapter is a discussion on how positive references to drinking in popular culture are normalizing drinking. Alcohol depictions in mass media are ubiquitious. Postmodern world is a world of images. Our identities and desires are manipulated by the images we come across everyday. Positive portrayal of drinking has serious repercussion on gender relations in a patriarchal society. Drinking when alligned with concepts of power, masculinity, sex and celibrityhood further bolsters gender inequalities. The libertine rake of twenty first century is a 'wild', 'adventurous' and 'carefree' man. Advertisements of alcohol brands extoll the adjectives like adventurous, carefree, reckless, wild, raw. These advertisements are consumed by audiences repeatedly which results in perpetuating such adjectives as norms. Being wild and carefree is translated as being irresponsible. The line between reality and constructed reality blurrs. Alcohol dependance becomes 'natural' whereas taking responsibilities of family members becomes an exception. The neagative aspect of alcoholism such as alcohol dependance, alcohol abuse, hangover, organs damage, diminished cognitive ability and domestic violence instigated by alcohol dependance are rarely depicted in music videos, movies, songs, TV serials and advertisements. One way of countering the negative effects of glamorization of drinking practice while treating alcoholics is narrative therapy. Narrative therapy works by enabling the patients to construct empowering life narratives about themselves thereby making them responsible for their life. It aims at giving them a sense of control.

The present discussion is divided in two parts. First part has two sections: Positive Portrayal of Drinking in Popular Culture and Violence, Alcoholism and Gender Binaries. First part elucidates critically how normalization of drinking entails violence and gender inequalities. The second part of the chapter has two sections: Alcoholism and Narrative Therapy, and Conclusion. This section includes case study of an alcoholic person and his treatment through narrative therapy.

POSITIVE PORTRAYAL OF DRINKING IN POPULAR CULTURE

> Sex and drugs and rock and roll
> is all my brain and body need
> They will try their tricky device
> trap you with the ordinary
> get your teeth into small slice
> the cake of liberty.
> (Ian Drury, Sex and Drugs and Rock and Roll)[1]

The lyrics of the song by Ian Drury are symptomatic of the glamour associated with drinking alcohol in popular culture. Television screens, print and social media offer a plethora of images which portray consumption of alcohol as a 'cool' practice. Drinking as portrayed in movies comes with its own paraphernalia. A man clad in elite apparels sitting in a posh restaurant with a glass of whisky and grooving to the tunes of loud music with scantily clad women hovering about him is the stereotype of a postmodern rake. In popular culture drinking is a personality trait common to all protagonists who go on to achieve great heights in life. In such a scenario alcoholism becomes a glamorous practice. Whereas side-effects of alcoholism in real life such as liver failure, alcohol abuse and alcohol dependence are obliterated. The culture starts imbibing the practices promoted by mass media. Drunkenness becomes a done thing. Expressing love and dancing under the influence of alcohol becomes a romantic practice. The signs of power in popular culture comprises of luxury, excessive indulgence in drinking and sex. Such life is the life of ecstasy and liberty. People who live a responsible life are often seen as mediocre. Excessive drinking is a sign of extremities and extremity is an integral part of a heroes' temperament. Celebrity lifestyle as represented in movies, songs and magazines is about opulence. Drinking the most expensive wine is emblematic of their vast fortune. Due to deluge of references in media, drinking is emerging as a social activity. TV programs often use alcohol as a catalyst to social gathering and celebrations. Almost every great event and its celebration in the program's narrative includes direct or indirect references to drinking. Hero under the influence of alcohol exhibiting extraordinary confidence in matters of sex and romance is a common scene on TV and in movies. Drinking becomes a source of Dutch-courage instigating romantic and sexual encounters. Drinking establishments, wine and beer store and hangovers are used as the background to introduce as well as bring characters together. Such portrayal of alcohol consumption leads to normalization of alcohol consumption (Amanda Atkinson, Gill Elliott et.al).[2]

VIOLENCE, ALCOHOLISM AND GENDER BINARIES

On the other hand drinking and driving, domestic violence and alcohol abuse are seen as exceptional cases. According to a report published by WHO across all cultures there exists a strong link between interpersonal violence and alcoholism.[3] Drinking results in less self-control as well as diminished cognitive ability. The ability to process received information also suffers that is why most people resort to violence when confronted. Diminished cognitive ability also makes drunken person prone to risky situations as they fail to perceive warning signs. Moreover, people who suffer violence also resort to alcohol for coping with violence. Thus a circle of violence and alcoholism is established.[3] Alcohol dependence is a grotesque fact that makes developing countries further financial impoverished. In most of the domestic violence cases reported in India alcohol dependence is the top most cause of violence. Dutch-courage as depicted in movies and television serials does not stop at romance. In a study conducted by McClelland *et al.*[9], it was found that the men under the influence of alcohol had fantasies of domination as compared to sober men.[7] The negative aspect of Dutch-courage in real life often results in intimate partner violence and sexual violence. Some other studies by Leonard and Quigley, Mc Kinney *et al.*[7,8] also found that partner violence episodes were more cruel when one of the partner was intoxicated. Reality is replaced by representation. Such phenomenon is called Simulacra and Simulation. The terms were propounded by French philosopher Jean Baudrillard.[4] According to Baudrillard capitalistic post-modern societies live in ecstasy of information. He questions the originality of information provided by media. Images are everywhere in our culture. Baudrillard sees images as a reflection of reality. Such perception of images is the first stage of representation. In the second stage the image obscures reality but still has some resemblance to it. At the third stage the final demolition of the relation between image (sign) and reality occurs and simulation takes place. At this stage images represent a reality which does not exist at all. Image pretends to be an authentic copy of something which has no original. There remains simulation only. Baudrillard writes: to stimulate is not simply to feign...feigning or dissimulation leaves the reality intact...

whereas simulation threaten the difference between real and imaginary.[4] Real is substituted by the sign of real. In the absence of an original the sign starts dictating perceived reality and images become the lens through which members of society see and interact with each other. Furthermore, according to Baudrillard the confusion and blurring of reality and imitation has another implication as well. Mass media platform such as television and internet manipulate their users' desire. By promoting the products through images and commercials which fool viewers into believing it to be an essential necessity of their life they aim at creating a pseudo- need for the product advertised. Aging is a natural phenomenon but airbrushing age from women's face is a routine when it comes to women's magazine. According to Dalma Heyn, the editor of a women's magazine, the effect of airbrushing the age is clear: "By now readers have no idea what a real woman's 60 year old face looks like in print because it's made to look to 45. Worse, 60-year-old readers look in the mirror and think they look too old because they are comparing themselves to some retouched face smiling back at them from a magazine" (Wolf,83).[10] Staying young is normal, aging is abnormal. Similarly, high end alcohol brands aim at associating masculinity with drinking. A famous Indian whisky brand has the motto 'Men will be men', another advertisement ends with the lines- it's your life make it large. Success, power, masculinity; all these qualities in real life has nothing to do with alcoholism. But commercial advertisements manipulate peoples' perception of a successful man. It is embedded in their psyche that in order to be successful and look powerful they have to indulge in so called masculine activities and one of them is alcoholism.

An identity is a role-playing. It is a performance. Our popular culture is offering images which are implicitly changing the paradigm of masculinity. This new masculinity is widening the chasm between gender roles as the figure promoted by popular culture in music videos and movies is of a man who is carefree, wild, adventurous and aberrant: someone who pretends to be 'himself' (JackDaniels' advertisement ends with the message be yourself). Due to the courtesy of such advertisement and stereotypes most of the men try to be carefree, wild and adventurous. They lead a decadent life. At this juncture Simulacrum and reality collide thereby bringing havoc on the personal and professional life of pseudo-heroes off TV screen. Being carefree is interpreted by most of the viewers as being irresponsible and insensitive to their wives' and children's' needs. Consequently, family for people suffering from alcoholism becomes a hurdle which prevents them from fulfilling their dream role. Such attitude towards family entails domestic violence and seperation. Alcoholism along with other ailments of post-modern world is a deep rooted psychological problem. Between identity and the stage lies reality: latent but profound.

It is interesting to note how many magazines for male and female readers subtly reinforce gender roles. These magazines often portray drunk women as 'easy lay'. Their presence in a 'male territory' such as bar, along with alcohol consumption is inferred as unfeminine. They are seen as 'modern' women open to random sexual encounters. Yet again the world is painted in black and white while classifying women through gendered lenses. Either they are 'sluts' who frequent pubs and bars or they are self-abnegating mothers who stay at home and take care of their families.

In most of the magazines for female readers one comes across articles which list negative effects of drinking on women's health and appearance. Most common listed side-effects are premature aging, sterility, hair-loss, under eye dark circles and glow less skin. Role of drinking act as a means of social interaction and making influential contacts is emphasized in magazines for men. The gender binaries which associate culture and public sphere with man can be seen at work. On the other hand same gender binaries align women with body and home. Thus very implicitly media indulges in gender injustices and inequalities.

ALCOHOLISM AND NARRATIVE THERAPY

In the first part of the chapter I elucidated how alcoholism is being depicted as an integral part of luxurious successful life. The modern libertine hero has its root in seventeenth century Restoration period in the literary history of England. Following lines by the John Wilmot, the iconic libertine figure of restoration age are evident of libertine hero's decadent and irresponsible life:

> I Rise at Eleven, I Dine about Two,
> I get drunk before Seven, and the next
> thing I do,
> I send for my whore, when for fear of a clap
> I spend in her hand , and I spew in her Lap.
> (John Wilmot, Regime de Vivre)[5]

Non conformity, excessive drinking and whoring were the sure signs of libertine heroes. Restoration plays in England attributed celebrity hood to such personalities. The presence of alcoholic irresponsible Casanova was visible on the English stage in nascent form. The ghost of 'Be Yourself' had arrived. On the other hand reality hit John Wilmot with full force. Gilbert Burnet wrote about John Wilmot.

For five years together he was continually drunk...which led him to do many wild and unaccountable things.

At the age of 33 John Wilmot died of STDs and syphilis. His death is an example of a bitter end due to uncritical adherence to libertine ethos.

Libertine model of existence along with postmodern market driven economies are able to influence peoples' attitude towards alcoholism by portraying alcoholism as a means to get recognized and accepted in social circle of power and festivities. Being alcoholic is translated as being modern, panache. It's an epicurean practice of an elite life. To cure such distorted perception of reality psychotherapy can be very useful. A form of psychotherapy is narrative therapy. The therapy works by helping the patient to construct a new and empowering narrative about their life and themselves. Narrative therapy claims to be a social justice approach seeking to challenge dominant discourse which shape peoples' lives in destructive ways. The propounder of narrative therapy were Michael White and David Epston. The narrative therapy works on the principle that personal narrative formed by a person about his/her life shape their identity. Another important aspect of this therapy is that it gives a sense of agency to the patient. The patient feels powerful as he/she takes control of the trajectory of their life narratives. They aspire to become better and more responsible. The methodology of narrative therapy can be best substantiated by the example of a case study conducted by Dr Kaminsky, Stanley Robinowitz and Riva Kasan titled 'Treating alcoholism through Narrative Approach'.[6] The case study is about Ron, a 28 year old university educated man married to a nurse. Due to excessive drinking his personal and professional life goes for a toss. He looks for acceptance and approval in family as well as workplace. When he is not accepted and his behavior is censored by people around him he becomes violent and abusive. The psychiatrist choses to cure his patient using narrative therapy and suggests Ron to write a novel where he himself is the hero of the novel. Ron starts to write the novel and the psychiatrist takes care of the formal and structural aspect of the novel whereas content is formulated by Ron alone. Gradually

Ron merges his life into novel's narrative and starts to see himself in new light. As a hero he strives to become more self-disciplined and responsible. Rather than emulating prevalent discourses about alcoholism dictated by popular culture he becomes conscious of the damaging effects of alcohol on his life. He realizes that in real life one lives and cares for others. Only beasts live in a carefree manner as they live to eat and sleep. When such realizations dawn upon him he abstains himself from alcohol and becomes a family man. After eight months of follow up Ron is still abstinent and responsible.[6]

CONCLUSION

The positive stereotypes of alcoholic man in popular culture is endorsing the consumption of alcohol. They do so by subtly aligning power, prestige, manhood and success with drunkenness. Viewers should be made aware that a drunken disciplined hardworking man is a contradictory term. It is a chimera which exists in realm of virtual world. A successful man is a responsible, focused and disciplined man who is accountable for his every action. TV screen and life are poles apart. Empowering life narratives have the capacity to subvert distorted and misguiding paradigms therby bridging the gap between word and world.

ACKNOWLEDGMENTS

Author thanks Dr. V.K. Shanwal (Gautam Buddha University) for the guidance and providing insightful perspectives. His expertise on the subject opened new avenues of interest in interdisciplinary studies.

REFERENCES

1. Ian Drury. 'Sex and Drugs and Rock n Roll'. Stiff Records, 26 August **1977**.
2. Amanda Atkinson, Gill Eliiott, Mark Bellis, Harry Sumnall. Young people, alcohol and the media. Www.jrf.org.uk, September **2011**.
3. World Health Organisation, WHO Policy Briefing **2006**.
4. Baudrillard, Jean. Simulations, Semiotext(e), **1983**.
5. John Wilmot, 2nd earl of Rochester. Regime de Vivre. https://en.m.wikitionary.org/wiki/ Talk: punk

6. David Kaminsky, Stanley Robinowitz, Riva Kasan. Treating alcoholism through narrative approach. Canadian Family Physician, vol 42 April **1996**.
7. Leonard, K.E., and Quigley, B.M. Drinking and marital aggression in newly weds: An event –based analysis of drinking and the occurrence of husband marital aggression. Journal of Studies on Alcohol and Drugs.
8. McKinney, C.M., Caetano, R.., Rodriguez, L.A., Okoro , N. Does Alcohol involvement increases the severity of intimate partner violence? Alcoholism: Clinical and Experimental Reaearch, 34: 655-8. **2010**.
9. McClelland, D.C., Davis, W.N., Kalin, R.., and Wanner, E. The drinking man: Alcohol and human motivation. Free Press,New York **1972**.
10. Naomi Wolf. The Beauty Myth. Vintage Books, Great Britain **1991**.

Editors' Note

Portraying the alcoholics as hero or person doing extraordinary tasks in different media like literature, movies, tv, radio or other popular media bring direct influence on society towards encouraging such substance abuse like alcoholism. The psychological therapy by narrating better consequent life for alcohol free living bring healing healthier life for alcoholics and society.

❑❑❑

13

Alcoholism Among Adolescents and Juvenile Delinquency

Annie Khanam (Singh)* **and Subhasis Bhadra****

Abstract

Alcoholism is one of the most prevalent public health issues among adolescent and young adults. Most of the cases of Juvenile delinquency raised in the current scenario are one of the consequences of alcoholism. A repeated pattern in drinking behavior, which is termed as binge drinking associates with many health issues. Problems like liver sclerosis, sexual dysfunction, fetal alcohol syndrome, alcohol poisoning and cardiac diseases are all results of excessive intake of alcohol. A report by the World Health Organization provides with the statistics which confirms that about 2.5 million deaths are caused due to alcohol inebriation worldwide. It is well evident that there is a strong correlation between alcohol and delinquent behavior. Juvenile delinquency and addictive behaviors have run hand in hand, further giving birth to major social problems. This chapter focuses on the efforts that are continuously being made worldwide to address the issue. It states the need of comprehensive treatment strategies that take into account the causes and effects of excessive alcohol

* Department of Psychology and Mental Health, School of Humanities & Social Sciences, Gautam Buddha University, Greater Noida, Uttar Pradesh, India

** Department of Social Work, Central University of Rajasthan, Ajmer, Rajasthan, India

consumption. Life skills education training is such a well-researched training method for enhancing the positive behavior among the vulnerable populations, likes alcoholics. This chapter explores on these two aspects, taking into account the use of alcohol among juvenile delinquents, and bringing out novel ways of decreasing this problem through life skills training as a part of school and college education.

Keywords: Alcohol abuse, Adolescents, Alcoholism, Juvenile Delinquency

INTRODUCTION

In the competitive life of the current worldwide scenario, the adolescent all over the world face many public health issues. Alcoholism comes up to be the most threatening and prevalent problem amongst the adolescent population. There have been various efforts being taken to decrease the occurrence of alcohol use among teens and adolescent populations.[1] The World Health Organization report of global status reflects that alcohol consumption has alarmingly increased in India from 2008 to 2012. The report states that 30% of the total Indian adolescent population consume alcohol.[2] Most of the cases of Juvenile delinquency have raised in the current scenario as one of the consequence of alcoholism. This chapter focuses on the efforts that are continuously being made worldwide to address this issue. It states the need of comprehensive treatment strategies that take into account the causes and effects of excessive alcohol consumption. Life skills education training is such a well-researched training method for enhancing the positive behaviours among the vulnerable populations, likes alcoholics. This chapter explores these two aspects, taking into account the use of alcohol among juvenile delinquents, and bringing out novel ways of decreasing this problem through life skills training as a part of school and college education.

Alcohol abuse in adolescents is a major issue that should be taken into consideration on priority basis all over the world. The challenges of present life styles create a background for adolescents to easily give into the temptations of alcohol and drug abuse. Failure of coping mechanisms and faulty communication increases risk of indulgence in such practices. All the social, personal and psychological developmental aspects are required to be focused to address the problem of alcohol adolescent abuse. Adopting a evidence-based therapeutic intervention instead of punitive approach leads to decrease in negative aspects and eradicates the problem like alcohol abuse and addiction from roots.

Defining and understanding the concept of Alcoholism

The journal of American Medical association defines Alcoholism as a chronic disease with psycho-social, genetic and environmental factors that play a vital role in its manifestation and development. World Health Organisation on the other hand takes into account the variable meaning of the term alcoholism, where it refers to it as chronic continuous drinking behaviour that impairs an individual's daily life, frequent alcohol abuse in spite of the adverse consequences.[3]

Research surveys indicate that there is a high rate of drinking behaviour in college going adolescents. This particular age group shows an increasing trend of alcoholism worldwide. These dangerous drinking practices further lead to other health compromising behaviours such as drug abuse, unhealthy sexual practices and diseases like tuberculosis and AIDS.[4] College students and young adults are becoming more prone to alcohol usage pertaining to the fact that they experience a transition phase due to the changes they go through in life at the time of entering school or college for higher learning. Most of them leave their families and start living independently, the reduced adult supervision and increased peer pressure leads to indulgence in habits like drug and alcohol abuse. Various social and environmental factors like college parties, social events also foster heavy usage of alcohol.[4] It can be clearly gathered Alcoholism is one of the most important issue that needs to be addressed on many levels as it targets the most important part of our World's population. It is difficult to define and analyse the term alcoholism, as it takes into account a wider aspect of human behaviour. It is important to understand all the possible causes and effects of alcohol abuse to eradicate it.

The Diagnostic Statistic Manual Criteria of Alcohol use Disorder

Alcohol use disorder is diagnosed as chronic relapsing disease that is marked by excessive alcohol use, uncontrollable alcohol intake and suffering from negative thoughts and negative emotional state, when an individual is not under alcohol's influence. To be diagnosed with Alcohol use disorder, a criteria outlined by Diagnostic and Statistical Manual of Mental Disorders (DSM) should be met. A person who meets any two of the eleven criteria mentioned within the period of 12 months are considered to be abusing alcohol. Larger the number of criteria's are met, severe the problem becomes. A study conducted in 2015 in U.S stated that 16 million people in the United States had alcohol use disorder.[5]

Epidemiological research findings indicate a disturbing trend of alcohol use in adolescent population. Youth mortality has resulted due to these dangerous drinking practices. The data indicates constantly increasing rates of alcohol usage through drinking practices like binge drinking and daily drinking. These practices have surfaced as major contributors to youth mortality. Suicides, road rage accidents are all results of alcohol abuse. Besides the youth themselves, their families are troubled and they miss the important part of their developing life in school and college. Alcohol consumption disrupts the life of youngsters in all its aspects.[4] The findings further indicate that both males and females have an almost equal rate of alcohol abuse.[6]

EFFECTS OF ALCOHOL ABUSE

Co-occurrence of few common additional health problems is seen alongside alcohol abuse of youngsters. These problems prove to be equally a menace to the healthy development of adolescent population all over the world. Tobacco use, Risky sexual behaviour, Drug abuse are the commonly seen issues that come up as sister issues of alcohol abuse.[7] Other Adverse effects Include: Alcohol poisoning, Academic failure, Fatal injuries, Violent behaviour including assaults and unintended pregnancies, Sexually transmitted diseases. The worst scenario may include HIV/AIDS, property damage, criminal activities that may risk the future of the young people involved.[7]

ROLE OF SOCIETY AND MEDIA

The cultural aspects and the symbolic myths that are used by media in advertisements of alcohol are also discussed widely. These directly influence the consumption of alcohol by the adolescent population. Warning related to alcohol consumption and smoking at the beginning of movies in theateres is a common practice, while on the contrary in the movies, the actors are shown smoking and consuming liquor as a normal practice. An adolescent mind comes across such contradiction and their thinking is affected deeply. In this way, society by practising such contradictory ideologies paves way for alcohol abuse and experimentation by youth. Their sensitive growing mind is unable to restrict itself from the attractive suggestion able media promotions. The contradictory factors like loose social structure and lack of law enforcement particularly leads to firm base of alcoholism and early exposure to drugs in adolescent population.[8]

Role of Familial factors

These risk factors include:

1. Childhood abuse and maltreatment by parents
2. Substance and alcohol abuse by parents
3. Level of education of parents
4. Parent Child relationship
5. Familial socio-economic status
6. Emotional Abuse
7. Social risk factors
8. Deviant peer relationship
9. Bullying
10. Gang Affiliation[9]

Mistreatment, abuse and neglect of children or adolescents by parents or care givers have strong evident links to increased risk of alcohol and substance abuse. A study report by US department of health and human services suggests that 29% of adolescents who have experienced some kind of abuse and maltreatment in childhood are indulged in some kind of abuse.[10] Emotional child abuse can be defined as a situation where a child's intellectual and psychological functioning is hindered. The data provided indicated that emotional abuse can lead to proneness of alcohol abuse.[11] Peer influence and deviant peer relationship have a positive relation with alcohol and substance abuse.[11] An adolescent forms an association with a peer group either to gain popularity or affiliation of a gang. The influence of peers on adolescent substance use often exists in the form of deviant peer relationships.[12] Research has shown that deviant peer relationships are positively associated with adolescent substance use.[11]

According to the National Institutes of Health bullying has been described as a series of interactions where a group or an individual verbally or physically abuses and assaults a victim who they perceive to be weak.[13]

In bullying both the perpetrator and the victim have been found to have an increased risk of mental health disorders and alcohol and substance abuse.[14] Gangsare usually defined as group of three or more people that are characterized by criminal behaviour. There have been found a positive association in literature, between Gang affiliation and alcohol abuse.[15] There is a sense of appeal in gang behaviour that attracts the adolescents to get affiliated with the gangs. It is the peer pressure that works in the excessive alcohol use within the gangs.[16]

Besides the above mentioned social and familial factors, there can be a few individual factors that are found to be responsible for excessive alcohol usage in adolescent population. These include Psychological and mental health issues like Depression, Attention deficit hyperactivity disorder (ADHD) and Post traumatic stress disorder.[9] A meta-analysis of thirteen studies have indicated that youth suffering from ADHD are more susceptible to develop substance abuse disorders and alcohol abuse during adolescent or adulthood.[17] Research has indicated a comorbidity of alcohol and substance abuse with depression are common in adolescents. These are found to be interlinked.[18] Depressed adolescent are at a higher risk of excessive alcohol use.

JUVENILE DELINQUENCY AND ALCOHOL ABUSE

Juvenile delinquency can be broadly defined as a term used for adolescents or children who commit crimes. Juveniles are defined as those people who haven't reached adulthood or the age of majority.[19] There are many reasons associated with delinquent behaviour. A significant aspect that leads us to establish a relation between Delinquent behaviour and alcohol abuse can be the present societal scenario that challenges adolescent population to the levels where their skills are tested on the paradigms of social and personal structures. Social adjustment is the key to decrease stress. By adolescence, youngsters require to master a broad array of skills that are required to achieve conventional goals in our society. These important skills include interpersonal skills (e.g., socializing and getting along with others, forming personal and intimate relationships), academic skills and work skills. Failure to acquire these skills affects the social adjustment of the adolescent. The literature associating survival skill deficits with delinquent adolescents suggests that, when most of the adolescent population is unable to match the expectation they end up feeling useless and depressed. This makes them vulnerable to all kinds of deviations like alcohol abuse which further leads to juvenile delinquency.[20]

ESTABLISHING A RELATION BETWEEN DELINQUENT BEHAVIOUR AND ALCOHOLISM IN ADOLESCENTS

Underage drinking can be considered a delinquent activity. Adolescents who engage in underage drinking are putting up themselves at risks like that of getting abused and assaulted. Youngsters often differ in their thought patterns than adults. They easily experiment and take risks. In this way they easily involve themselves in antisocial activities, which include excessive alcohol use and drug abuse. They become victims of crime once marked by such an event in life, makes them vulnerable to delinquent behaviour and adult criminality.[21]

Adolescent alcohol abuse raises a chance of a wide variety of mental health issues. Depression, suicidal tendencies, low self-esteem and loneliness are few major issues that every adolescent has to deal with. In order to avoid stress, youngsters start taking alcohol and drugs, this paves way for all the other related health risk behaviours. Mental health issues develop rapidly in youth with alcohol abuse disorder than the normal counterpart population.[22] Alcohol abuse involves risk to areas of critical development of adolescents. Physical and emotional health is essential for youths to develop and mature into behaviourally healthy individuals. When this developmental process is hindered, it results into disturbed adolescents that result into alcohol abuse and delinquent behaviour at many instances. Researches have indicated that even mild involvement in alcohol abuse at school or college level can significantly disturb the development process.[23] Alcohol abuse disrupts functioning at school and increases psychological and interpersonal impairment. An adolescent becomes vulnerable and thus, gets involved into secondary problem behaviours like that of delinquency due to alcohol abuse.[24]

There are many concerns related to adolescent alcohol abuse and involvement in the risk behaviors. It enhances the chances of serious problems in areas critical to development. For youth to mature into successful adults, clearly they need not only to be physically and emotionally healthy, but also to become successful in domains essential for their roles as adults. Alcohol use during adolescence disturbs normal life style of an adolescent in school and at work. It further surfaces interpersonal and psychological impairment. It completely changes the trajectory of adolescent's development and reduces potential healthy adult functioning.

PREVENTIVE METHODS AND INTERVENTIONS FOR DECREASING ALCOHOL ABUSE

The best way to devise a preventive measure for adolescent drinking problems is to relate to it on its developmental aspect. There is a need to apply the whole system approach to take into account the risk factors and the protective factors. These factors range from genetic to social, personality traits to environmental. In order to resolve the issue, an overview concentrating on both individual and social factors has to be taken up.[25] The Periods of rapid transitions, when an adolescent goes through a social or cultural transition which also strongly influence the biology and behaviour of the adolescent. This transition phase can be considered as best to intervene through various corrective measures in order to address the alcohol abuse problem in adolescents.[26] Interventions targeting this critical phase can be of great help in addressing this issue at its root. The alterations made at this phase can decrease the risk of engaging in alcohol abuse later in life.

US department of health and human services in its article proposes for two forms of Intervention methods first being the environmental factors and second being the individual factors

ENVIRONMENTAL LEVEL INTERVENTIONS

Raising the Prices of Alcohol Beverages

There is a strong link between decreased alcohol consumption with increased price of alcohol beverages. Adolescent population is seen to mostly abuse the alcohol or drugs that are easily available and affordable. Increased prices can directly prevent excessive alcohol usage in adolescents.[27]

Increasing the Minimum Legal Drinking Age

Maximum countries in world have a minimum legal drinking age of 21. India through all its states vary from 18 to 25.[28] There is an utmost need to increase the legal drinking age. This can work as the most simple and effective measure to decrease alcohol abuse in adolescent population. The estimates of National Highway Traffic Safety Administration provide the information that such law has prevented more than 21000 traffic deaths.[29]

Forming Zero Tolerance Laws

Law enforcement related to the drinking age or drinking and driving should be followed seriously. The loopholes that create space for leniency should be addressed to prevent excessive alcohol abuse in adolescent population.[30]

Individual-focused interventions include:

School-Based Prevention Programs

Alcohol abuse is a problem that needs to be addressed at the earliest possible stage. Intervention programmes designed to be followed at schools can be of great help to make the children understand the consequences of alcohol abuse and its adverse effects in their later lives. Earlier such programmes used to be informative but recent scenario includes practical approach that include social and individual factors to frame norms that can help children resist the pressure of drinking and substance abuse. These programs offer information on interactive and development appropriate information which includes peer aspects and components that lead to drinking through peer pressure. An approach of teachers training has also been included as a fresh component to decrease the risk of alcohol abuse peer-led components, and provide teacher training.[31]

Family-Based Prevention Programs

Including parents and family members can be of immense help in decreasing alcohol abuse.[32] An adolescent learns both on individual to social level to abstain from alcohol use. A constant drugs and alcohol free environment in the family and society encourages the juveniles and young generation to abstain from use of drugs and alcohol. The parents and senior family impact the learning behaviour of young ones. Further, senior members can be friendly in understanding the problems of young ones and guide them or serve helping hand to young ones which ultimately influence the socio-psychological behaviour leading to avoidance of drugs and alcohol. Monitoring by family members can reduce likelihood of engaging in alcohol abuse.[33]

INSTITUTION BASED CORRECTION AND REHABILITATION PROGRAMS

There are corrective measures that are institution based. These include families and communities as a part of their applicable approach in eradicating alcohol abuse and other problem behaviours that are related to it.

Multisystemic Therapy

It is one of the effective approach that addresses antisocial behaviour of the adolescents who abuse alcohol and drugs. Adolescents participate in intensive treatment that is often given in the natural environment of either their homes, school or a correctional facility. It specifically reduces adolescent alcohol and drug abuse.[34]

Multidimensional Family Therapy

It caters to the problem behaviour of adolescents who abuse alcohol and drugs. It is a multi-dimensional correctional approach. It includes both individual sessions and interactive sessions with family. It works within the network of individual, family, peer and community. Its overall approach addresses the issue on the whole basis for long term results.[35]

Brief Strategic Family Therapy (BSFT)

It focuses family interactions considering them as causes or enhancers of alcohol abuse and other problem behaviours like conduct issues, oppositional behaviour, delinquency, aggression and risky sexual behaviour of adolescents. This therapy approaches the family system and monitors the trigger factors associated with problem behaviours. This therapy takes up a flexible approach in a broad range of family situations. It can be practiced at mental health clinics, social service settings and in family environment as well.[36]

Functional Family Therapy (FFT)

It is a treatment based approach which focuses on family systems. This therapy targets the problem behaviours associated with family dysfunctional interaction patterns. Adolescents who belong to broken and alcoholic's families are the major focus of this therapeutic approach. It aims at enhancing parenting skills, conflict resolution and communication between adolescent and the family members. It is effective in resolving conduct and delinquency problems in adolescents.[37]

LIFE SKILLS AND ALCOHOL ABUSE PREVENTION

Life skills education works on the principle of ten generic skills. A combination of these skills enhances psycho social competence of an individual. It can act as an ideal stress management program. It is easy in practice and follows a pattern of participatory and experiential learning. It aims at developing knowledge and attitudes along with skills. It works on enhancing communication skills, interpersonal relations and decision making abilities.[38] The Life Skills Training (LST) program is an effective primary prevention program for adolescent drug and alcohol abuse that focuses on these factors as well as enhancing social and personal competence skills. Life skill education can be used as an effective intervention to enhance attitudes and skills of adolescents. It targets evaluation of stress and identifies best coping methods suitable to the set ups like correctional facilities.[39] It is a widely used training module that has a broad applicability. It has proved its successful implication in a wider perspective all over the world. A Model given in a WHO document,[40] shows the place of life skills as a combination of motivating factors of knowledge attitudes and values and positive health behaviour, which contribute in prevention of mental health problems. It can be applied to enhance psychological health and wellbeing in organisational set ups.

Preventive approaches like life skills training majorly focus protective factors associated with initiation of drug and alcohol use in adolescents. This program trains an adolescent in skills that are most important in building resistance for problems like alcohol abuse and delinquent behaviour.[41] Short term effects have been witnessed in few studies that provide an evidence of effectiveness of life skills training in reducing alcohol abuse.[42] In other studies with a follow up of 5 to 6 years, long term effects of life skills intervention training on reducing alcohol abuse in its participants is clearly evident. The intervention group was found to be engaged in 50% less binge drinking relative to controls at the 1- and 2-year follow-up assessments.[43] Life skills programs are designed in such a way that they come up as an effective tools to combat alcoholism and youth substance use.[44]

Life skills education training can be of immense help in increasing and maintaining psychological health of adolescents in school, college and correctional settings. Life skills education can act as an important tool to equip adolescents to negotiate and arbitrate challenges that they face in life situations. It can enable a productive participation within the institutes and society.

CONCLUSION

In the present scenario, alcohol abuse and its sister issues like drug addiction and delinquent behavior in adolescent population has become an eye catching issue all over the world. Adolescence is the most sensitive part of an individual'slife. An individual faces a lot of pressure and conflicts at this phase. In due course majority of adolescents become vulnerable and indulge themselves into faulty practices that risk their future and present. This along with it generates secondary risk behaviors that contribute to form a vicious cycle of addiction, crime and risk behaviors. An adolescents falls prey to this circle and their life is adversely affected. There is a contradictory aspect in relation to the laws related to alcohol and liquor consumption in India. Different states have different age range for buying and consumption of alcohol. This difference creates a loophole in the system. So it becomes difficult for the authorities to check illegal alcohol consumption and control excessive intake in the underage population. In the present scenario, there is a need to approach this issue with a broader outlook and at early stage in schools and colleges. There is a need to address the leglislative aspect of alcohol consumption in India with strictness. There are various correctional and rehabilitative approaches present that work to eradicate these issues. Life Skills is one of such intervention program that can be used both at institutions and at individual level.[45]

Life skills training reduces substance and alcohol use and related behaviours such as aggression, withdrawal, truancy, and stealing in adolescents. Life skills uses participatory learning methods that initiate a positive behavioural change, which eventually leads to decrease in habits like alcohol abuse. As it is evident that besides high use of alcohol among adolescents, there are additional health compromising behaviours like drug abuse, risky sexual practices and teen pregnancies. Life skills targets these secondary problems that affect the lives of adolescent population, Research data has indicated effectiveness of life skills education training program in addressing mental health issues and behavioural problems on a wide platform. There is a need to set up life skills based intervention program in schools and colleges, along with correctional facilities for juvenile delinquents. Social policies and Intervention programs in school and college campuses should incorporate various training and informative methods to effectively modify alcohol abuse and its immediate health risk behaviours.

REFERENCES

1. Johnson, L. D., O'Malley, P. M., & Bachman, J. G. (**2003**). Monitoring the Future National Survey Results on Drug Use. National Institute of Drug Abuse.
2. World Health Organisation. (**2014**). Global status report on alcohol and health.
3. Morrow, D. (2017). The Alchoholism guide. Retrieved from www.the alchoholism-guide.org.
4. Windle, M. Alcohol Use among Adolescents and Young Adults. **2003**.
5. National Institute of Acohol Abuse and Alcoholism. (2017, june wednesday). Alcohol Use Disorder. Retrieved from www.niaaa.nih.gov
6. World Health Organisation. (2015). Mental health. Retrieved January, 2017, from http://www.who.int/topics/mental_health/en/
7. Singh, J., Chhikara, B.S. Comparative global epidemiology of HIV infections and status of current progress in treatment. *Chemical Biology Letters*, **2014**, 1(1), 14-32.
8. Pechanskyl, F., Szobot, C. M., & Scivoletto, S. (**2004**). Alcohol use among adolescents: concepts, epidemiological characteristics and etiopatogenic factors. *Official J. Brazillian Psychiatric Association.*
9. Whitesell. M, Bachand. A, Peel. J, & Brown. M. Familial, Social, and Individual Factors Contributing to Risk for Adolescent Substance Use. *J Addict.*, **2013**.
10. U.S. Department of Health & Human Services. (2013, july). What Is Child Abuse and Neglect? Recognizing the Signs and Symptoms. Retrieved from Child Welfare Information Gateway
11. T. E. Duncan, S. C. Duncan, H. Hops. The effects of family cohesiveness and peer encouragement on the development of adolescent alcohol use: a cohort-sequential approach to the analysis of longitudinal data. *J. Studies on Alcohol*. **1994**, 588-599.
12. E.M. Trucco, C.R. Colder, J.C. Bowker, W.F. Wieczorek. Interpersonal goals and susceptibility to peer influence: risk factors for intentions to initiate substance use during early adolescence. *J. Early Adolescence*. **2011**, 526-547.
13. U.S National Library of Medicine. (2017, june). "Bullying: Medline Plus. Retrieved from http://nlm.nih.gov
14. T.R. Nansel, M. Overpack, R.S. Pilla, W.J. Ruan, B.S. Morton, P. Bullying behaviors among US youth: prevalence and association with psychosocial adjustment. *J. Am. Med.* Assoc. **2001,** 2094–2100.

15. Thornberry, T. P., Krohn, M. D., Lizotte, A. J., & Wierschem, D. C. The role of juvenile gangs in facilitating delinquent behavior. *J.Res Crime Delinq.* **1993,** 30, 55–87.

16. National Gang Center, (2012). Gang-Related Legislation: Colorado. Retrieved from nationalgangcenter.gov: http://www.nationalgangcenter.gov/Legislation/Colorado.

17. Wilens, T. E., Martelon, M. K., Clancey, B. B., Bateman, C., Fried, R., Carter, P., & Biederman, J. Does ADHD predict substance-use disorders? A 10-year follow-up study of young adults with ADHD. *J. Am. Acad. Child Adolesc. Psychiatry*. **2011,** 543–553.

18. P, W. c., Hoven, N., Okezie, C., Fuller, C. J., & Cohen, P. Alcohol abuse and depression in children and adolescents. *J Child Adolesc Subst Abuse.* **2008,** 51–69.

19. United Nations. (**2003**). World youth report; Global situation of young people. United Nations Publications.

20. Vitaro, B. F. Influence of Deviant Friends on delinquency: searching for moderator variables. *J Abnorm Psychol.* **2000**, 313-325.

21. Drug and alcohol rehab, Asia. (2017, june thursday). Delinquency and Substance Abuse. Retrieved from alcoholrehab.com

22. Lilienfeld, S. O., Waldman, I. D., & Israel, A. C.A critical examination of the use of the term and concept of comorbidity in psychopathology research. Clinical Psychology-Science and Practice.*Clin. Psychol.***1994**, 1, 71-83.

23. Brown, S. A., & Tapert, S. F. (2004). Health Consequences of Adolescent Alcohol Involvement. In R. J. O'Connell, Reducing Underage Drinking. National Academic Press.

24. Rohde, P., Lewinsohn, P. M., Seeley, J. R., & Brown, R. A. Natural course of alcohol use disorders from adolescence to young adulthood. *J Am Acad Child Adolesc Psychiatry*, **2001,** 83–90.

25. Sroufe, L. A., & Rutter, M. (1984). The domain of developmental psychopathology. Child Development, 17–29.

26. Masten, A. S. (2004). Regulatory processes, risk, and resilience in adolescent development. Annals of the New York Academy of Sciences, 310–319.

27. Leung, S. a. (1993). My kingdom for a drink. . . . ? A review of estimates of the price sensitivity of demand for alcoholic beverages. Economics and the Prevention of Alcohol-Related Problems, pp. 1–31.

28. Banerjee, R. (2016). 6 Bizarre State Laws Regarding Liquor Consumption in India. Retrieved from www.indiatimes.com

29. National Highway Traffic Safety Administration (NHTSA). (2003). Traffic Safety Facts 2002: Alcohol. Washington DC: National Center for Statistics & Analysis.

30. Jones, R. K., & Lacey, J. H. (2001). Alcohol and Highway Safety 2001: A Review of the State of Knowledge. Retrieved from National Highway Traffic Safety Administration, 2001.

31. National Institute on Alcohol Abuse and Alcoholism. Interventions for alcohol use and alcohol use disorders in youth. *Alcohol Res Health.* **2004/2005,** 28, 163–174.

32. Steinberg, L., Fletcher, A., & and Darling, N. (1994). Parental monitoring and peer influences on adolescent substance use. *Pediatrics*. **1994**, 93, 1060–1064.

33. Spoth, R. L., Clair, S., Shin, C., & Redmond, C. Long-term effects of universal preventive interventions on methamphetamine use among adolescents. *Arch Pediatr Adolesc Med.* **2006**,160, 876-882.

34. Henggeler, S., Halliday-Boykins, C., Cunningham, P., Randall, J., Shapiro, S., & Chapman, a. J.E. Juvenile drug court: Enhancing outcomes by integrating evidence-based treatments. *J Consult Clin Psychol*. **2006**, 42–54.

35. Liddle, H. A., & Houge, A. Multidimensional family therapy for adolescent substance abuse; E. F. Wagner, & H. B. Waldron Ed; Innovations in Adolescent Substance Abuse Interventions London, **2001**;pp. 227-261.

36. Santisteban, D., Suarez-Morales, L., Robbins, M., & and Szapocznik, J. Brief strategic family therapy: Lessons learned in efficacy research and challenges to blending research and practice. *Family Process*, **2006,** 259-271.

37. Waldron, H., Slesnick, N., Brody, J., Turner, C., & and Peterson, T. Treatment outcomes for adolescent substance abuse at 4- and 7-month assessments. *JCCP*, **2001** 802–813.

38. UNICEF. (2012). Global Evaluation of life Skills Education Program. New York: United Nations Children's Fund.

39. Whybra, L. (2016, March). Finding better evidence for "evidence-based" programs. Retrieved from www.preventionaction.org

40. World Health Organisation. (2017). Adolescents: health risks and solutions. Retrieved from ww.who.int: ww.who.int/mediacentre/factsheets/

41. Botvin, G. J., & Griffin, K. W.Life skills training as a primary prevention approach for adolescent drug abuse and other problem behaviors. *Int J Emerg Ment Health.* **2002,** 41-47.

42. Botvin, G. J., Griffin, K. W., Diaz, T., & Williams, I. Preventing binge drinking during early adolescence: One- and two-year follow-up of a school-based preventive intervention. *Psychol Addict Behav*, **2001,** 360-365.

43. Spoth, R., Redmond, C., & and Shin, C. (2001). Randomized trial of brief family interventions for general populations: Adolescent substance use outcomes 4 years following baseline. *JCCP*.**2001**, 627–642.
44. Giannotta, f., & Weichold, K. Evaluation of a Life Skills Program to Prevent Adolescent Alcohol Use in Two European Countries: One-Year Follow-Up. *JRPCS Springer*. **2016**, 607–624.
45. Singh, A., & Bhadra, S. Life Skills Education (LSE) for Juvenile Delinquent: Developing a Behaviour Health Promotional Model. *Artha Journal of Social Science*. **2015**, 19-31.

Editors' Note

Alcoholism in young generation is prevalent and increasing diligently assisted by social reflections of character along with many other factors from family, peer-group and society. A control stringent measure set by society and organizations form essential part of combating the menace of alcoholism in young population.

❑❑❑

14

Impact of Alcoholism on Various Aspects of Wealth Management

Shweta Anand*

Abstract

It is well known by past research findings that Alcoholism leads to loss of jobs implying loss of salary. Also it leads to troubled marital life leading to higher rate of divorce which implies maintenance/settlement charges. Alcoholism also burns a hole in the pocket which leaves lower residual income for investments towards financial goals. Risk to health goes up and so does the cost of medical and life insurance. This study has tried to analyze the impact that Alcoholism has on these as well as various other aspects of Wealth Management.

Keywords: Alcoholism, Wealth Management, Investment Portfolio, Financial Goals

INTRODUCTION

Alcoholism and its impact on the various social aspects have been studied in the past. The human beings spends his childhood and youth to learn the skills that will help him earn a livelihood. Each person has financial goals that he strives to achieve once he starts earning. Hence, for a human being since all efforts are directed towards earning, saving and achieving

* School of Management, Gautam Buddha University, Greater Noida, India.

financial aspects it was analyzed, the financial inclusion aspects was also taken into account.[1] It was analysed if the habit of Alcoholism had any impact on achieving financial goals.

Wealth Management is the bigger umbrella which has various aspects.[2] The Various aspects of Wealth Management as being analyzed in this chapter are:

1. *Budgeting:* All sources of income constitutes the Revenue Inflow. All expenses are money outflow. The residual amount left each month is the investible amount. A part of these is the amount which get invested towards achieving financial goals each month.
2. *Financial Goal Setting:* This implies goals that need finances to be achieved. Becoming famous or a good human being is a generic goal. However, buying a house is a financial goal and one has to consiously invest towards achieving the same.
3. *Risk Appetite:* The ability and willingness to take risk related to returns while investing money explains the Risk taking Appitite of an individual.
4. *Planning an ideal Investment Portfolio:* There are various investment options available such as Shares, Bonds (like NSC, NSS, Fixed Deposits, Infrastructure bonds etc.), Gold, Property, Cash (including Savings bank balance, Money market investments). A portfolio is like a pie chart representing combinations of these investment options. (Example: 30% in Shares, 50% Fixed deposit, balance cash)
5. *Risk Management:* Risk to regular investing towards achieving financial goals can come from sudden medical emergencies, accidents, loss of life of bread earner, etc. These risks can be covered or managed using Insurance Policies of Mediclaim and Life Insurance. Two social aspects, Job continuity (loss of income) and Divorce (payment of settlement) were also analysed under the umbrella of Risk Management as they too have an negative impact on overall Wealth Management. There are however no insurance policies in India to cover these risks.

This chapter concentrates on how achieving Wealth Management gets disrupted or disturbed or delayed due to the habit of alcoholism.

Moreover the overall negative savings that are caused by Alcoholism is also analyzed.

RESEARCH METHODOLOGY

Personal interview using semi structured questionnaire was done of about 50 regular drinkers who were either married or divorced and the data collected personally[3] was analyzed against expectaions as well as existing benchmarks. Only those respondents were interviewed who consumed alcohol on three or more days per week. All respondents interviewed were men and bread earners in the family. Data was asked of the household unit of the respondent. Household Unit is defined as Self, Spouse and Kids. This implies that data related to total income, expenditure, savings, investments, portfolio etc of household unit was asked for.

Also, a focus group discussion was done with Investment Experts and Insurance Agents. Also, various websites and related research papers were analyzed and studied.

The following Hypothesis were tested

- Alcoholism has no Impact on family budget.
- Alcoholism has no Impact on Financial Goal Setting
- Alcoholism has no Impact on Risk Appetite
- Alcoholism has no Impact on planning an ideal Investment Portfolio towards meeting the Financial Goals.
- Alcoholism has no Impact on Risk Management

DATA ANALYSIS

Data Analysis of the various aspects of Wealth Management[4] which were analysed after normalization of data[5,6] and detailed below :

Impact on Budgeting

Hypothesis Tested: Alcoholism has no Impact on family budget.

The respondents were asked 'What amount of your monthly budget gets spent on expenses related to your habit of Alcoholism -0-5%, 5-10%,10-15%,15-20%,20-25%,25-30%, more than 30%?' Most respondents were spending in the range of 20-25%,25-30%. Note, Monthly Income – Monthly Expenditure = Maximum amount available towards investments.

This implies that an increase of 25% (average) in expenditure leads to 25% lesser amount available to invest towards achieving financial goals.

The overall impact on savings is approximately 25% or quarter of the earnings. Hence, it can be concluded that Alcoholism has a significant Impact on family budget.

Impact on Financial Goal Setting

Hypothesis Tested: Alcoholism has no Impact on Financial Goal Setting

On being asked to list down their financial goals which they would like to achieve, most respondents were planning for next goal which was buying a car or buying a house. Long term goals such as higher education of child, marriage expenses of children, medical contingency fund and retirement fund were not being planned for.

Hence, a holistic view of all short term goals and long term goals was not being considered. Instead just the next one, short term goal was the guiding light for investing.

Since a secure long term objective view was not seen in any respondent it can be concluded that Alcoholism has a impact on confidence level and hence a significant Impact on Financial Goal Setting.

Impact on Risk Appetite

Hypothesis Tested: Alcoholism has no Impact on Risk Appetite

A standard scale was used to find out the Risk Appetite score of respondents. The results showed that the average risk appetite for each age group of respondents was lower than the corresponding standard scores expected for the said age groups. On probing further the respondents revealed that the habit of Alcoholism was impacting efficiency at work. This implies lower annual performance bonus, slower promotions and overall a risk of being shown the door or retrenchment. Since most respondents felt the risk of job stability they were not too comfortable with high risk investments.

High Risk: High Return. There is a direct relationship between risk embedded in the investment option and the expected returns from it. For example shares of a company may give very high or very low returns. Since the expected return is volatile they are considered as very risky investments. However, literature review reveals that on annualized year-on-year basis the shares as a asset class gives highest return on investment.

But with Alcoholism leading to lower risk appetite – the money that would be invested would be invested on low risk-low return investments such as Fixed Deposits, Government Bonds.

Hence, Alcoholism has significant Impact on Risk Appetite. It reduces substantially the appetite to take risk as per ones age and life stage. This implies that lower income would be generated from the investments.

Impact on Planning an Ideal Investment Portfolio

Hypothesis Tested: Alcoholism has no Impact on planning an ideal Investment Portfolio towards meeting the Financial Goals.

A portfolio consists of investments in various asset classes such as 1. Fixed Income Securities, 2. Domestic Shares, 3. Foreign Shares, 4. Gold, 5. Property and 6. Cash.[7] Respondents were asked in which of the above asset classes the current net worth of the family was invested. They were asked to mark the approximate percentage of total investments made as a household unit in various asset classes. Since risk appetite was seen as low the impact on investment pattern was also similar. Almost 80-90% of the portfolio was invested in safe to moderately safe investment options such as Government Bonds, Fixed Deposits, Debt Mutual Funds, Gold and Property.

At a young age '80 less age' is ideal amount to be invested in shares. This can be done either directly or through share broker or indirectly via mutual funds. However, based on age and life stage the actual amount invested in shares against expected ideal investment was almost nil or negligible.

This implied that Alcoholism was discouraging the respondent from harnessing all the high risk but high return investment options available in the market. Not having an ideal Investment Portfolio Mix was delaying the meeting of the families Financial Goals.

Hence, Alcoholism has significant Impact on planning an ideal Investment Portfolio towards meeting the Financial Goals. Thus, investments as a independent source of income was not generating the maximum potential returns that an ideal portfolio mix as given age and life stage could have generated.

Impact on Risk Management

Hypothesis Tested: Alcoholism has no Impact on Risk Management

Risk is inherent in every aspect of life. Nothing is certain in today's life. There is enough documentary evidence to prove that Alcoholism increases the following risks substantially:

1. Risk of bad health and resultant medical costs.
2. Life expectancy of alcoholics is lower.
3. Job continuity and performance is poor
4. Probability of broken marriages and divorce.

Risk Management aspect 1, Risk of bad health and resultant medical costs can be covered by buying General Insurance policies of mediclaim.[8] However the premium charged if insured is an alcohol consumer is substantially higher. Data analysis of premium calulation tables evailable with Insurance agents were analysed. It revealed that respondents were paying 15-20% more than other insured of their age for the same insurance cover but if they were non-drinkers.

Insurance company can technically **refuse** to give mediclaim policy if medical reports show high levels of Alcoholism.[9] 18% of the respondents had been refused Mediclaim policy based on medical reports.

Moreover, in case of accidents if the FIR or any other evidence proves that it was a case of 'Drink and drive' than the medical expenses **claim will be rejected**. Out of 50 respondents, two had faced such accidental claims and in both cases it was refused for this reason.

Risk Management aspect 2, Life expectancy of alcoholics is lower, however, the risk of the household unit of loosing the bread earner of the family can be covered using Life Insurance.[10] In life insurance policies too premium charged if insured is an alcohol consumer is substantially higher. Data analysis revealed that respondents were paying 15-20% more than other insured of their age but non-drinkers.

Insurance company may **refuse** to give Life Cover Policy if medical reports show high levels of Alcoholism. 20% respondents had been refused Life Insurance policy based on Medical Reports.

Moreover, in case of accidental deaths if the FIR or any other evidence proves that it was a case of 'Drink and drive' than the insurance **claim will**

be rejected. Since data was not taken of such cases further analysis of such cases was not possible.

Risk Management aspect 3, Job continuity and performance is poor and cannot be covered via any general insurance policy. Such policies can be seen in other countries but an analysis of availability of such policies drew a blank in Indian context.[11] Respondents had revealed that the habit of Alcoholism was impacting their efficiency at work. This implied to them lower annual performance bonus, slower promotions and overall a risk of being shown the door or retrenchment. Since most respondents felt the risk of job stability and there was no insurance policy to cover this risk, this risk was to be borne by the respondents.

Risk Management aspect 4, Alcoholism increases the probability of broken marriages and divorce.

Of the 50 respondents chosen at random, 9 were divorced or on final stages of being divorced. Hence the rate was 18%.

Five respondents spoke of marital discord and fights which was rooted in the habit of Alcoholism. In case the scenario did not change they felt it could lead to separation/divorce.

The reason why this personal aspect was being analyzed is because divorce leads to payment of alimony and maintenance money which is agreed upon and paid lump sum and/or as a monthly installment thereafter. This further reduces the amount available to invest for future goals. Of the 9 divorcee respondents 60% of them had taken loans including expensive personal loans on credit cards towards paying the settlement amount. This was leading to negative savings due to EMI payments each month.

Hence, it can be concluded after analyzing the following aspects related to Risk Management

Risk of bad health and resultant medical costs is high,

Life expectancy of alcoholics is lower and cost of insurance cover is higher,

Job continuity and performance is poor and

Probability of broken marriages and divorce runs high.

Risk of bad health and early eventuality goes up. Insurance is either costlier or refused. Risk of divorce runs high and leads to further negative savings due to settlement costs. Hence, Alcoholism has a very significant and negative impact on Risk Management aspect of Wealth Management.

FINDINGS

The findings that there was an increase of 25% (average) in expenditures which lead to 25% lesser amount available to invest towards achieving financial goals shows that Alcoholism has a significant Impact on family budget. The findings that a holistic view of all short term goals and long term financial goals was not being considered showed that financial investing was not being done prudently. Instead just the next one short term goal was the guiding light for investing.

The analysis showed that Alcoholism was having a negative impact on confidence levels related to job security and hence a significant Impact on Financial Goal Setting. This implies that lower income would be generated from the investments.

Alcoholism showed significant Impact on Risk Appetite. It reduces substantially the appetite to take risk. This implied that Alcoholism was discouraging the respondent from harnessing all the high risk but high return investment options available in the market. Not having an ideal Investment Portfolio Mix was delaying the achievement of the Financial Goals of the household unit. Hence, Alcoholism has significant Impact on planning an ideal Investment Portfolio towards meeting the Financial Goals.

Alcoholism has shown a very significant and negative impact on Risk Management aspect of Wealth Management. Risk of bad health and resultant early eventuality goes up. Insurance is either costlier or refused by Life Insurance Companies. Risk of divorce runs high and leads to further negative savings due to settlement and maintenance costs which are unavoidable.

CONCLUSION

As concluded from literature review not much research has been done in the past on impact of Alcoholism on Wealth Management. The impact on various aspects of Wealth Management has been studied in this research from respondents who were regular drinkers or Alcoholics. The impact on all aspects of wealth management which were analyzed was significant and negative. Hence, it can be concluded that the habit of Alcoholism is not good for the financial health of a household unit.

ACKNOWLEDGMENTS

The author is grateful to Gautam Buddha University for encouragement and condusive academic environment towards working on this study.

REFERENCES

1. N. Kumar. Financial Inclusion and its Determinants: Evidence from India. *J. Financial Economic Policy*, **2013**, 5(1), 4-19.
2. V. Chauhan, V. Chaudhary. Discussion Paper on Internet Banking: Challenges and Opportunities in Indian Context. *J. Management Sci. Technology*, **2015**, 2(3).
3. T.-H. Kim, H. White. On more robust estimation of skewness and kurtosis. *Finance Research Letters*, **2004**, 1(1), 56-73.
4. J.R. Hosking. L-Moments: Analysis and estimation of distributions using linear combinations of order statistics. *J. Royal Statistical Society. Series B (Methodological)*, **1990**, 52(1), 105-124.
5. J. M. Bland, D.G. Altman. Statistics Notes: Cronbach's Alpha. *BMJ: British Medical Journal*, **1997**, 314(7080), 572.
6. J.A. Gliem, R.R. Glem. Calculating, Interpreting, and Reporting Cronbach's Alpha Reliability Coefficient for Likert-Type Scales. Midwest Research to Practice Conference in Adult, Continuing, and Community Education. **2003**.
7. M.A. Canela, E.P. Collazo. Portfolio selection with skewness in emerging market industries. *Emerging Markets Review*, **2007**, 8(3), 230-250.
8. https://www.insurancepandit.com/(aggregator of all Indian Insurance Policies) retrieved on 10th January 2017.
9. https://www.irdai.gov.in/ IRDA (Insurance Regulatory and Development Authority of India) retrieved on 15th October 2016.
10. https://www.licindia.in/ (Life Insurance Corporation of India) retrieved on 30th Dec 2016.
11. https://www.policybazaar.com/ (aggregator of all Indian Insurance Policies) retrieved on 1st January 2017.

Editors' Note

Alcoholism lead to a number of financial implications for affected person and associated family members, which indirectly indicate the instability pattern of livelihood in the society. The poor are affected more, lead to job lose, poor health of affected person with burden on health management system, and degrading social behavioural set up.

Alcohol free society can bring better financial growth and wealthier populace.

❑❑❑

15

Chemical Therapeutics for the Treatment of Alcoholism

Brijesh Rathi* and Poonam**

Abstract

Alcoholism treatment involves various therapies including psychological counselling, body message, herbal medicine, and allopathy (chemical drugs). The chemical drugs used for the treatment of alcoholism are very diverse structurally and have different drug targets in the body. The drugs approved and under investigation for the treatment of alcoholism have been discussed in this chapter for pharmacological properties, potential of application, side effects and chemical structural design.

INTRODUCTION

Alcoholism also known as alcohol use disorder, is a very common neuropsychiatric disease that has extensive health and socioeconomic impacts. The chronic alcohol consumption enables numerous medical indications *viz.* addiction and damage to the functioning of organs.[1] Notably, there is no magical medication available that can eliminate the desire to drink alcohol except counselling and rehabilitation therapy. However, there are several therapeutic drugs have been developed to treat the alcoholism, which are used for the additional treatment in some of the more severe cases. Advanced research in neurobiology suggested the

*Department of Chemistry, Hansraj College, University of Delhi, Delhi-110007 India
**Department of Chemistry, Miranda House, University of Delhi, Delhi-110007 India

expansion of medicines to treat alcoholism by modifying the activity of the specific chemical messengers (i.e., neurotransmitters). Few drugs were purposely designed and developed to lower the cravings for alcohol. In the brain, the tailored activity of neurotransmitters is crucial to treat the alcoholism. Food and Drug Administration (FDA) approved few drugs (i.e., antabuse,_naltrexone,_acamprosate) for the specific treatment of alcoholism. These medications are helpful for a person to concentrate on the work of recovery and ease the long-term effects of alcohol withdrawal. The most capable new medications is acamprosate, which seems to reduce the force of craving after a person has stopped drinking. However, several other drug molecules targeting neurological disorders have been employed for the treatment of alcoholism[2,3]; further research is essential to regulate their effectiveness and how medicines interact with different psychosocial factors. The details of therapeutic drugs (Figure 1) used for the treatment of alcoholism are described in this chapter.

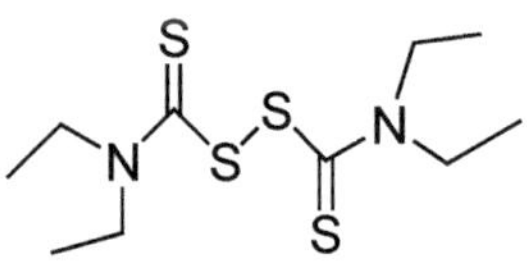

Antabuse
(Disulfiram)

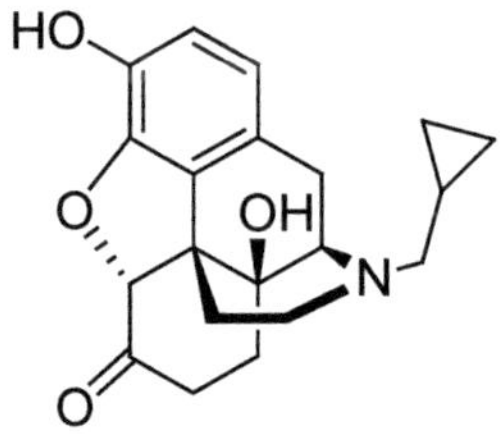

Naltrexone

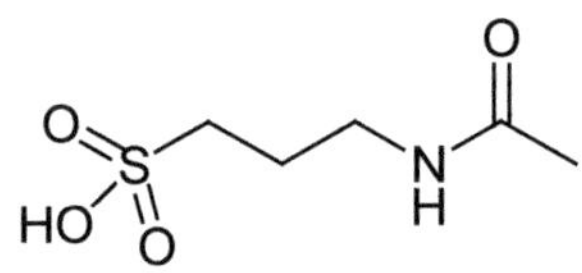

Campral
(Acamprostate)

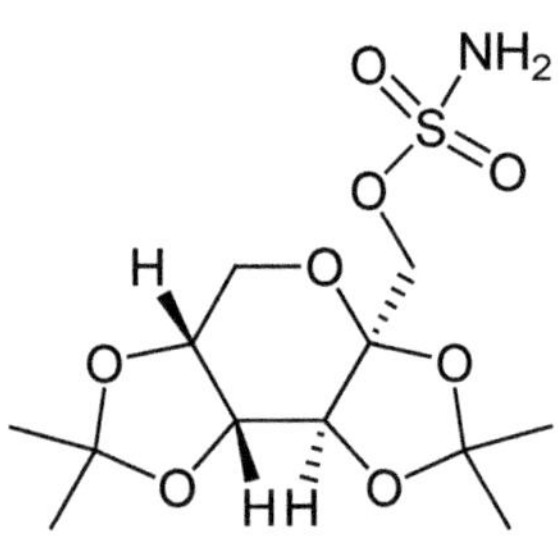

Topamax
(Topiramate)

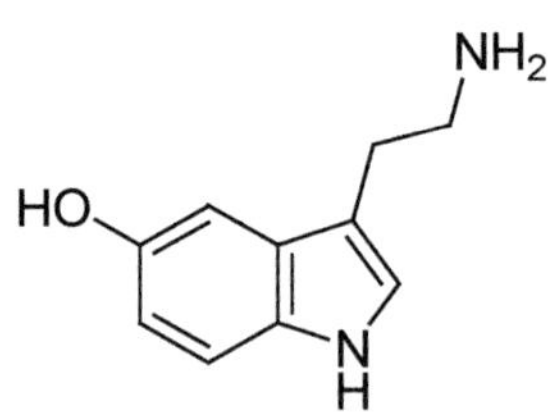

Serotonin

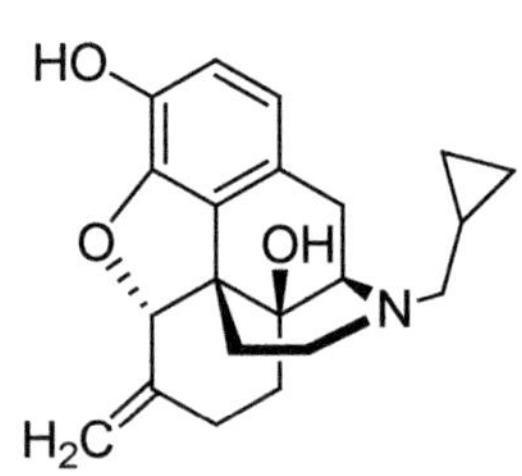

Nalmefene
(Nalmetrene)

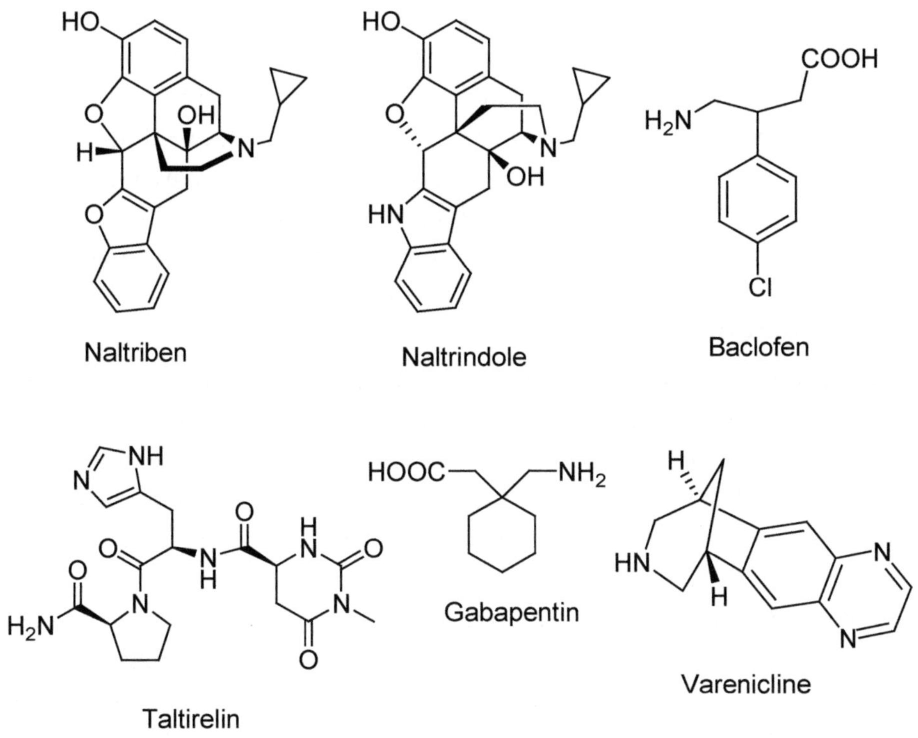

Fig. 1 Chemical structure of the therapeutic agents used for alcoholism.

Chemical Drugs used for Alcoholism

Following are the synthetic chemical drugs that are used in the management of alcoholism.

1. Antabuse

Antabuse, known as disulfiram is being employed as therapeutic drug for the treatment of alcoholism since more than 50 years. This is one of the oldest drugs for the treatment of alcoholism. Danish and his co-workers in 1948, investigated the intolerance to the alcoholic beverages after ingestion of disulfiram known as tetraethyl-thiuramdisulfide (T.E.T.D.).[4] This drug functions by intervening with the capacity of body to absorb alcohol, particularly by dropping the production of an enzyme that would otherwise allow the body to absorb an alcohol breakdown product, acetaldehyde. When enzyme is not available to break it down, acetaldehyde shapes up in the body after even little alcohol is consumed resulting in flushing, nausea, and palpitations.[4] Antabuse is used to treat chronic alcoholism. The main limitation associated with antabuse is the unpleasant side effects that will occur if people consume alcohol while taking antabuse. Even small amounts of alcohol can produce unpleasant symptoms while antabuse is present in the body. Allergic reaction to antabuse: hives; difficult breathing; swelling of the face, lips, tongue, or throat are common. The craving cannot be destroyed by antabuse. The effectiveness of antabuse is highly increased when its use is monitored either by clinical experts or family members.

2. Naltrexone

Naltrexone, classified as an opioid antagonist, is a synthetic analog of oxymorphone helping to reduce the feeling of craving for alcohol.[5] Naltrexone is helpful in reducing the liking that alcoholics obtain from drinking and the cravings that induce them to consume more alcohol. All these processes are achieved by blocking the receptors in the brain for endorphins, the proteins formed by the body that help to elevate the mood. Naltrexone can be taken as a once-daily pill or in a lately accepted once-monthly in injection form. It has been observed that initially, after one or two drinks, an alcohol consumer instead of discontinuing shows more craving for alcohol. They become eager to have more drinks that leads to addiction. Naltrexone pauses that encouraging reaction loop. After having the medical treatments with naltrexone, after one or two drinks person do not sense to have more drinks. From the clinical studies, oral naltrexone was revealed to decrease the amount of relapses to heavy drinking.[5]In comparison studies, the patients who consumed a placebo (dummy pill), the alcoholics treated with naltrexone had 36% fewer heavy drinking events over a three-month period.[5]Now a days, naltrexone is offered in a once-monthly injectable form called Vivitrol, which is advantageous over the daily intake of the drug.

3. Acamprosate

Acamprosate also called as campral (3-Acetamidopropane-1-sulfonic acid), is classified as an opioid antagonist. Acetaldehyde dehydrogenase inhibitor, disulfiram, yields several unpleasant effects when consumed along with alcohol, experiential confirmation favoured the effectiveness of acamprosate and naltrexone in treating alcoholism.[6,7] Acamprosate reduces the craving for alcohol intake and also aids to improve some of the side effects of alcoholism. Although, the detailed mechanism of action of acamprosate is not completely investigated. Several experimental data indicated, it functions through the modulation of the glutamatergic N-methyl-D-aspartate (NMDA) receptor.[8] A recent controversial investigation suggested the mechanism of action of acamprosate, which specify the calcium portion of the molecule as the only effectivecomponent.[9] Acamprosate is well tolerated non-toxic therapeutic drug having diarrhoea and headaches as the adverse effect. Acamprosate is recommended as three 333 mg tablets thrice a day in patients with a body weight above 60 kg and two tablets two times a day in patients with a bodyweight below 60 kg.[6]

The NMDA-receptor antagonist, acamprosate acts to lower the craving intensity after drinking cessation, particularly when the patient is exposed to the conditions linked with previous alcohol use, where the threat of relapse is highest.[10] Acamprosate was observed to lower the consumption of alcohol in rats without intervening with total fluid and food intake.[3]Few investigations have directly evaluated effect of acamprosate on alcohol-related behaviours in humans. Nevertheless, a magnetic resonance imaging (MRI) study displayed reduced glutamatergic efficacy in certain brain regions in humans following acamprosate administration, supporting its potential intreatingalcoholism.[11] Clinical investigation played a major role in supporting the effectiveness of acamprosate for the treatment of alcoholism.

4. Topamax.

Topamax also known as topiramate is approved therapeutic drug for the treatment of epilepsy[12] and migraine.[13] This drug has been examined as an effective treatment for a plethora of psychiatric and internal medicine conditions,[14] including metabolic complaints such as diabetes mellitus and obesity,[15,16] anxiety-related disorders such as post-traumatic stress disorder (PTSD)[17]and impulse dyscontrol-related disorders etc.[18] The neuropharmacological activities of topiramate involve enabling of the inhibitory activity of GABA (Gamma-aminobutyric acid) at its non-benzodiaze-pine receptor and decrease of the glutamate excitatory action at the alpha-amino-3 hydroxy-5 metylisoxazole-4 propionic (AMPA) receptor and the kainate receptors.[19,20] This drug is anticipated to decline the reward effects of alcohol intake by decreasing the mesolimbic cortical action of dopamine.[21,22] Topiramate has ~80 % bioavailability and a half-life of 19–23h. The drug achieves its maximum concentration between 1.3 and 1.7h post-ingestion and its steady-state plasma concentration in about 4 days.[23] Topiramate was first suggested as a treatment for alcohol abuse, however, it is not specifically approved by the FDA for the treatment of alcohol use disorder. Topiramate failed to prove superiority in reducing craving for alcohol.[24]

5. Serotonin

Selective serotonin reuptake inhibitors (SSRIs) are the treatments that intervene the removal of serotonin from the synapse following release of the neurotransmitters. In humans and animals, intake of alcohol has been shown to alterserotonin-receptor action, and preliminary studies have suggested that administration of SSRIs can decrease alcohol intake in animals.[25]The stimulation of specific serotonin-receptor subtypes can inspire dopaminergic function in the nucleus accumbens (aportion of brain affected by many drugs of abuse and implicated in the process of reinforcement), hence contributing to the rewarding effects of alcohol.[2a]Nevertheless, the connection between serotonin-reuptake inhibition, food intake, and fluid consumption is complex.[26] Thus, the effect of SSRIs on alcohol drinking could be attributable to general decrease in consummatory behaviour. Serotonin is highly crucial for the regulation of various physiological functions, including body rhythms, sleep, and mood states, as well as appetitive and consummatory behaviors.[25] Out of fifteen known subtypes of the serotonin receptor, a few are highly valuable for the development of alcohol-use disorders through numerous communications with other neurotransmitter systems in the body. The potency of serotonergic agents in treating alcoholism is well investigated during last two decades.[24]

6. Nalmefene and its derivatives

Nalmefene, an opioid antagonist is known as nalmetrene, which is used mainly in the management of alcohol dependence.[27] It is an antagonist at mu- and delta-opioid receptor and a partly agonist at the kappa receptor. Initially in 1990s, nalmefene was approved in United States of America for the treatment of opioid overdoses. Nalmetrene is structurally similar to naltrexone, where ketonic group is substituted with methylene group. This drug offers several advantages such as more effective binding to the central opioid receptors, a higher bioavailability and the absence of a dose-dependent association with liver toxicity.[24] Moreover, the oral bioavailability of nalmefene is slightly higher (40 %) than that of naltrexone.[28] The toxicity of nalmetrene to the liver cells has not been reported.

Several investigations advocated that antagonists of the delta opioid receptor namely naltriben and naltrindole are capable to defeat alcohol intake in animals,[29] however, further animal and human studies are required to evaluate the actual potency. The benzofuran analog of naltrindole, naltriben is a competitive nonpeptide delta opioid antagonists, which is derived from naltrexone. Naltriben has similar effects to the more widely used delta antagonist naltrindole, but with different binding affinity.[30] Naltriben also functions as a κ-opioid agonist at high doses.[31]

7. Baclofen (Lioresal)

Baclofen is one of the recently studied drug evaluatedas potent in helping patients stay abstinent. This drug is a muscle relaxant and anti-spasmodic, and is presently being investigated in patients with alcoholic cirrhosis.[24]

8. Taltirelin (TA 0910)

Taltirelin is a novel thyrotropin releasing hormone (TRH) analog, which has been investigated to characterize the acute effect different doses on ethanol intake in rat models.[32] This drug was approved for use in human beings in Japan. Several investigations suggested that acceptance to the effects of TA-0910 on alcohol intake occurs and indicated dopamine participation in the mechanism of action of TA-0910 in falling alcohol intake in animal models.[28,32]

9.Gabapentin

Gabapentin drug is being used in the alleviation of somatic symptoms of alcohol withdrawal. In vitro and in vivo models of CNS hyperexcitability during alcohol withdrawal suggested similar protective effects of gabapentin. Recently, gabapentin was explored as the treatment of alcohol dependence by Paniand co-workers.[33]

10. Varenicline.

Varenicline is an approved drug for smoking treatment. This drug is currently marketed as Chantix. Recently, varenicline has been investigated as beneficial for alcohol disorders.[34] Varenicline's mechanism in nicotine dependence includes partial agonism of $\alpha 4\beta 2$ and full agonism of $\alpha 7$ nicotinic acetylcholine receptors positioned in the ventral tegmental part of the brain, therefore regulating the complete effect of exogeneous nicotine on dopaminergic pathways.[24]

COMBINATION THERAPY.

The applications of multiple therapeutic drugs working at various sites have been recognised as more effective treatment for alcoholism.[35] Two clinical investigations confirmed that a combination of naltrexone and acamprosate is more effective than either single drug.[36] The interactions between neurotransmitters indicated that the combination of therapeutic drugs could be a potential treatment of alcoholism. For example, the combination of naltrexone and acamprosate, naltrexone decreases the craving derived from alcohol's positive rewarding effects[5], acamprosate reduces craving associated with the period following acute withdrawal.[10] Hence, the combination of naltrexone and acamprosate makes a patient to withhold easily from alcohol and also might be helpful in preventing a "slip" from turning into a relapse. Several critical issues associated with medication combination, including optimal dosing and timing, duration of treatment, and management of potential adverse interactions are important to achieve the potency of the treatment. Besides, therapeutic drugs, cognitive behavioural therapy (a form of psychotherapy focusing on identifying and modifying negative thoughts and thought patterns) and motivational enhancement therapy are valuable for the treatment of alcoholism.

Conclusion

A number of chemical molecules have been evaluated for their potency as treatment of alcoholism and few have been approved for the management of alcoholism. The approved drugs are complex in structure and generally have different degree of side effects on the patients. A further new molecules need to be developed with better pharmacological profile for the management of alcoholism.

References.

1. R. Spanagel, F. Kiefer. Drugs for relapse prevention of alcoholism: ten years of progress. *Trends Pharmacol Sci.* **2008**, 29, 109-115.
2. a) B. A. Johnson, N. Ait-Daoud. Medication to treat alcoholism. *Alcohol Res Health.* **1999**, 23, 99-106 and references cited therein; b) R. M. Swift, Drug therapy for alcohol dependence. *N Engl J Med.* **1999**, 340, 1482–1490.
3. R. Z. Litten, J. Allen, J. Fertig. Pharmacotherapies for alcohol problems: A review of research with focus on developments since 1991. *Alcohol Clin. Exp. Res.* **1996**, 20, 859–876.

4. J. Hald, E. Jacobsen, V. Larsen. The sensitizing effect of tetra-ethylthiuramdisulphide (Antabuse) to ethyl alcohol. *Acta PharmacolToxicol.* (Kbh.), **1948**, 4, 285-296.
5. J. R. Volpicelli, A. I. Alterman, M. Hayasgida, C. P.O'brien, Naltrexone in the treatment of alcohol dependence. *Arch Gen* Psychiatry, **1992**, 49, 876–880.
6. S. Rosner, A. Hackl-Herrwerth, S. Leucht*et al.*Acamprosate for alcohol dependence. *Cochrane Database Syst Rev.***2010**,8, CD004332.
7. N. C. Maisel, J. C. Blodgett, P. L. Wilbourne *et al.*Meta-analysis of naltrexone and acamprosate for treating alcohol use disorders: when are these medications most helpful? *Addiction*,**2013**, 108, 275–293.
8. J. Littleton, W. Zieglgansberger. Pharmacological mechanisms of naltrexone and acamprosate in the prevention of relapse in alcohol dependence. *Am J Addict***2003**, 12, (Suppl 1): S3–S11.
9. R. Spanagel, V. Vengeliene, B. Jandeleit *et al.* Acamprosate produces its anti-relapse effects via calcium. *Neuropsychopharmacology***2014**, 39, 783–791.
10. R. Spanagel, W. Zieglgänsberger, Anticraving compounds for ethanol: New pharmacological tools to study addictive processes. *Trends inPharmacological Sciences* **1997***,* 18, 54–58.
11. N. Bolo, J. F. Nedelec, M. Muzet, P. De Witte, A. Dahchour, P. Durbin, J. P. Macher, Central effects of acamprosate: Part 2. Acamprosate modifies the brain in-vivo proton magnetic resonance spectrum in healthy young male volunteers. *Psychiatry Res.***1998**, 82,115–127.
12. J. A. French, A. M. Kanner, J. Bautista *et al.*Efficacy and tolerability of the new antiepileptic drugs II: treatment of refractory epilepsy: report of the Therapeutics and Technology Assessment Subcommittee and Quality Standards Subcommittee of the American Academy of Neurology and the American Epilepsy Society. *Neurology***2004**, 62, 261-1273.
13. R. G. Wenzel,K. Schwarz, R. S Padiyara. Topiramate for migraine prevention. *Pharmacotherapy* **2006**,*26*, 375–387.
14. G. Rubio, I. Martinez-Gras, J. Manzanares. Modulation of impulsivity by topiramate: implications for the treatment of alcohol dependence. J. Clin. Psychopharmacol,**2009**, 29, 584–589.
15. G. A. Bray, P. Hollander, S. Klein *et al.*A 6-month randomized, placebo-controlled, dose-ranging trial of topiramate for weight loss in obesity. *Obes. Res.***2003**, 11, 722–733.
16. K. N.Chengappa Roy, J. Levine, D. Rathore *et al.*Long-term effects of topiramate on bipolar mood instability, weight change and glycemic control: a case-series. *Eur. Psychiatry***2001**, 16, 186–190.

17. C. P. Alderman, L. C. McCarthy, J. T. Condon *et al.*Topiramate in combat-related posttraumatic stress disorder. *Ann.Pharmacother.***2009**, 43, 635–641.

18. S. L. McElroy, L. M. Arnold, N. A. Shapira *et al.*Topiramate in the treatment of binge eating disorder associated with obesity: a randomized, placebo-controlled trial. *Am. J. Psychiatry***2003**,160, 255–261.

19. M. Angehagen, L. Ronnback, E. Hansson *et al.* Topiramate reduces AMPA-induced Ca(2$^+$) transients and inhibits GluR1 subunit phosphorylation in astrocytes from primary cultures. *J. Neurochem.***2005**, 94, 1124–1130.

20. H. S. White, S. D. Brown, J. H. Woodhead *et al.*Topiramate modulates GABA-evoked currents in murine cortical neurons by a nonbenzodiazepine mechanism. *Epilepsia***2000**; 41 (Suppl 1): S17–S20.

21. B. A. Johnson, N. Ait-Daoud, F. Z. Akhtar *et al.*Oral topiramate reduces the consequences of drinking and improves the quality of life of alcohol-dependent individuals: a randomized controlled trial. *Arch. Gen. Psychiatry***2004**, 61, 905–912.

22. F. Weiss, L. J. Porrino. Behavioral neurobiology of alcohol addiction: recent advances and challenges. *J.Neurosci.***2002**, 22, 3332–3337.

23. B. A. Johnson, Ait-Daoud N. Topiramate in the new generation of drugs: efficacy in the treatment of alcoholic patients. *Curr. Pharm. Des.***2010**, 16, 2103–2112.

24. M. Soyka, M. Lieb. Recent Developments in Pharmacotherapy of Alcoholism, *Pharmacopsychiatry***2015**, 48, 123-35 and references cited therein.

25. D. M. Lovinger, Serotonin's role in alcohol's effects on the brain. *Alcohol Health Res. World***1997**, 21, 114–120.

26. K. Gill, Z. Amit, Serotonin uptake blockers and voluntary alcohol consumption. A review of recent studies. *Recent Developments in Alcoholism,* **1989**, 7, 225–248.

27. G. A. Mason, A. H. Rezvani, D. R. Grady, J. C. Garbutt, The subchronic effects of the TRH analog TA-0910 and bromocriptine on alcohol preference in alcohol-preferring rats: Development of tolerance and cross-tolerance. Alcohol. Clin. Exp. Res.**1994**, 18, 1196–1201.

28. K. Ingman, N. Hagelberg, S. Aalto *et al.*Prolonged central mu-opioid receptor occupancy after single and repeated nalmefene dosing. *Neuropsychopharmacology***2005**, 30, 2245–2253.

29. J. C. Froehlich, M. Zweifel, J. Harts, L.Lumeng, T. K. LI, Importance of delta opioid receptors in maintaining high alcohol drinking. *Psychopharmacology***1991**, 103, 467-472.

30. M. Sofuoglu, P. S. Portoghese, A. E. Takemori. Differential antagonism of delta opioid agonists by naltrindole and its benzofuran analog (NTB) in mice: evidence for delta opioid receptor subtypes. *J. Pharmacol. Exp. Ther*. **1991**, 257, 676-80.

31. P. E. Stewart, E. M. Holper, D. L. Hammond. Delta antagonist and kappa agonist activity of Naltriben: evidence for differential kappa interaction with the delta 1 and delta 2 opioid receptor subtypes. *Life Sciences*. **1994**, 55, PL79-84.

32. A. H. Rezvani, J. C. Garbutt, K. Shimoda, P. L. Garges, D. S. Janowsky, G. A. Mason, Attenuation of Alcohol Preference in Alcohol-Preferring Rats by a Novel TRH Analogue, TA-0910. *Alcohol. Clin. Exp. Res.***1992**, 16, 326-330.

33. P. P. Pani, E. Trogu, M. Pacini*et al.*Anticonvulsants for alcohol dependence. *Cochrane Database Syst. Rev*.**2014**, 2, CD008544.

34. B. L. Erwin, R. M. Slaton. Varenicline in the treatment of alcohol use disorders. *Ann. Pharmacother*. **2014**, 48, 1445–1455.

35. A. H. Rezvani, D. H. Overstreet, G. A. Mason *et al.* Combination pharmacotherapy: a mixture of small doses of naltrexone, fluoxetine, and a thyrotropin-releasing hormone analogue reduces alcohol intake in three strains of alcohol-preferring rats. *Alcohol Alcohol.* **2000**, 35, 76-83.

36. F Kiefer, K. Wiedemann,Combined therapy: what does acamprosate and naltrexone combination tell us? *Alcohol Alcoholism* **2004**, 39, 542-547.

Editors' Note

The alcoholism can be managed by various chemical drugs like Antabuse, Naltrexone, Campral. Though these being selected chemical drugs that find application in recovery of alcoholics, these have their own side effects. A very careful selection of drugs and doses has been warranted depending on physiological condition and addiction level of patient.

❑❑❑

16

Alcoholism: A Health and Social Evil

Dharam Pal Singh* and Meenakshi Sindoliya**

Since ancient times, the general conception is in favour of acceptance of alcohol consumption in Indian culture. In recent time, the things have changed into disaster as there is now serious problem arising due to alcohol abuse in India as compared to past. According to World Health Organization (WHO) in 2013, globally 139000 deaths were directly due to alcoholism. The report also revealed that more than 11% of Indians were consumers against the global average of 16%. The per capita consumption of alcohol in India has increased almost 38% in a decade from 1.6 liters in 2003 -2005 to 2.2 liters in 2010-2012. National crime records bureau (NCRB) released data related to alcohol and health analysis in the year 2013 says 15 people dies every day, or one in every 96 minutes due to alcohol related health problems. In the report it was mentioned that role of political support to crack downs against the use of alcohol was not implemented due to their opinion of the use of alcohol as a health problem not a moral one. As per the psychiatric diagnosis in 2013 alcohol abuse in which there is recurring harmful use of alcohol despite its negative consequences, it was reclassified as alcohol use disorder (Alcoholism) along with alcohol dependence, There are two types of alcohol abuse - those who have anti social and pleasure seeking tendencies and those who are anxiety ridden people who are able to go without drinking for long periods of time but are unable to control themselves once they starts.

*SRDW College, Kolsiya, Jhunjhunu, Rajasthan
**Mewar University, Chittorgarh, Rajasthan

As per the habit of drink there are two different categories of drinkers

Social drinkers: This type of consumers do not drink to get drunk and they obey certain kind of law while drinking, know when to stop.

Bing drinking is the category of drinkers usually gets four to five drinks in a single sitting.

DEFINITIONS

Alcohol: Ethyl alcohol or ethanol is an intoxicating ingredient found in beer, wine and liquor, alcohol is produced by the fermentation of the yeast, sugar and starches.

Alcohol abuse: Alcohol abuse is a pattern of drinking that result in harm to one's health, interpersonal relationship or ability to work.

Abuse: It is called abuse when the consumer fails to fulfill role obligations at work, school or home.

India is the third largest market for alcoholic beverages in the world. According to annual report Government of India, Ministry of food processing industries the demand for spirits and beers is estimated to be around 373 million cases. Consumption of alcoholic beverages in different part of the world is influenced by economic, social and religious traditions of countries. These differ significantly in the amount and type of alcoholic beverage consumed. India has largest youth population which is getting influenced by external factors and has started consuming alcohol at a much higher rate and at early age.[1]

Among elementary school children, exposure to beer commercials is related to beliefs about beer drinking and expectation to drink as adult.

The social, culture and economic growth of any society is generally determined by the degree of intellect development of its young generation.[3] It is the young generation who is responsible to eradicate poverty and to enable people to lead a better and healthier life. Since, young generation is the foundation of political, economic, technical, and social development. Their education is a supporting factor. Despite the great responsibilities of students, there are serious problems of drug abuse to throw their life into dangerous future of nation. The fact is that the young population is vulnerable social group which is exposed to alcohol abuse practices and causes disastrous effects.

Higher rate of alcohol addiction is a major problem in India. In Punjab, Haryana, Manipur, Rajasthan nearly 75% of its youth are severely addicted to alcohol either in form of beer or wine or whisky etc.[2]

ALCOHOL ADDICTION:

Alcohol addiction also known as alcoholism, is a disease that affects people of all walks of life. It is important to note that alcoholism is real disease it can cause changes to the brain and neuro chemistry, so a person with an alcohol addiction may not be able to control their action.

Alcohol addiction can show itself in a variety of ways. The severity of disease, how often someone drinks and the alcohol they consume varies from person to person; some people drink heavily, whole day while other drink and then stay sober for a while.

Regardless of how the addiction looks, someone typically has an alcohol addiction if they heavily rely on drinking and cannot stay sober for an extended period of time.

Symptoms of alcoholism:-

Drinking is a part of life of many people when is it common in society, it can be hard to tell the difference between someone who likes to have a few drinks now and then and someone with a real problem. Some symptoms are

- Increase quantity and frequency of use
- High tolerance for alcohol, or lack of "hangovers"
- Drinking at in appropriate time, such as first thing in the morning, or in work and religious places
- Wanting to be where alcohol is present and avoiding situations where there is none.
- Changes in friendship, some with an alcohol addiction may choose friend who also drink heavily
- Avoiding contact with loved ones
- Hiding along, or hiding while drinking
- Dependence on alcohol to function in everyday life
- Increase lethargy, depression, or other emotional issues
- Legal or professional problems such as an arrest, or loss of a job

As an addiction trend to get worse over time, it is important to look for early warning signs. If identified and treated early, someone with an alcohol addiction may be able to avoid major consequences of the diseases.

HEALTH COMPLICATIONS OF ALCOHOLICS:

Drinking too much on a single occasion or over time can take a serious toll on the health of individual. Alcoholics' major affected organs and associated diseases are:-

Brain: Alcohol interference with the brain functions, communication pathways and can affect the way brain looks and works. This disruption can change mood and behavior, and make it harder to think clearly and move with coordination.

Heart: drinking a lot over a long time or too much on a single occasion can damage the heart, causing problem including cardiomyopathy, arrhythmias, strock, hypertension.

Liver: Heavy drinking takes a toll on liver and can lead to a variety of problems and liver inflammation including steatosis or fatty liver, alcoholic hepatitis, fibrosis cirrhosis of liver.

Pancreas: alcohol causes the pancreas to produce toxic substances that can eventually lead to pancreatitis that prevents proper digestion.

Cancer: Drinking too much alcohol can increase risk of developing certain cancer of mouth, esophagus, throat, liver, pancreas and breast.

Effect on immunity: alcohol can weaken immune system, making the body virulent for other diseases chronic drinkers are more liable to diseases like pneumonia and tuberculosis than people those do not drink.

Alcoholism causes disorders such as ulcers, diabetes complications, sexual problems, birth defects, bone loss, vision problems.

Effect of alcohol on personality:

Alcohol affects every organ of the body, it is a central nervous system depressant. It is readily absorbed from the stomach and small intestine into the bloodstream, alcohol is metabolized by an enzyme CYP2E1 however the liver can only metabolize a small amount of alcohol at a time, leaving the excess alcohol to circulate throughout the body. The intensity of the effect of alcohol on the body is directly related to the amount consumed.

Some people react differently to alcohol than others. Individual reactions to alcohol vary, and are influenced by many factors such as Age, Sex, Race, Ethnicity, physical condition, amount of food consume before drinking, time of consumption of alcohol, use of drugs, family history of alcohol problems.

Alcohol withdrawal symptoms:

Alcohol withdrawal symptoms can result in following physical and psychological symptoms like insomnia, tremors, anxiety, digestive discomfort, loss of appetite, headache, excessive perspiration, palpitation, hallucination, seizures and delirium.

FACTORS RESPONSIBLE FOR ALCOHOL CONSUMPTION:-

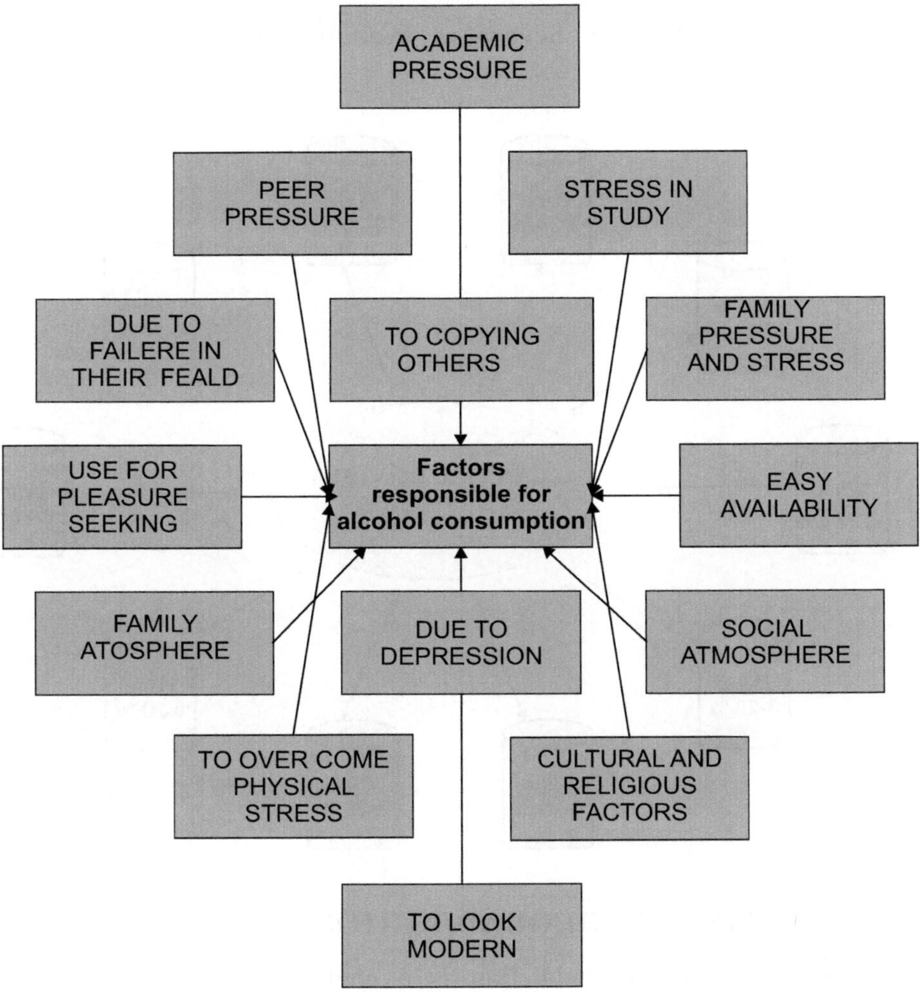

The causes of alcohol abuse are complex, alcohol abuse is related to economic and biological origins and is associated with adverse health consequences.

According to various studies conducted, the response of the adolescent towards alcohol is different. Attitude ranged of acceptance is casual approached, usually abuser does not know that he is suffering from which kind of disorder.

Generally the young people consider alcohol consumption as common part of normal life and it is glamorized to have alcohol. Many youngsters consume alcohol due to cultural influences.

Caste system in India also attributes to alcohol consumption and best exemplified by carstairs (1979) research conducted in Rajasthan.

A variety of **alcoholic beverages available** are given in following diagrammatic scheme:-

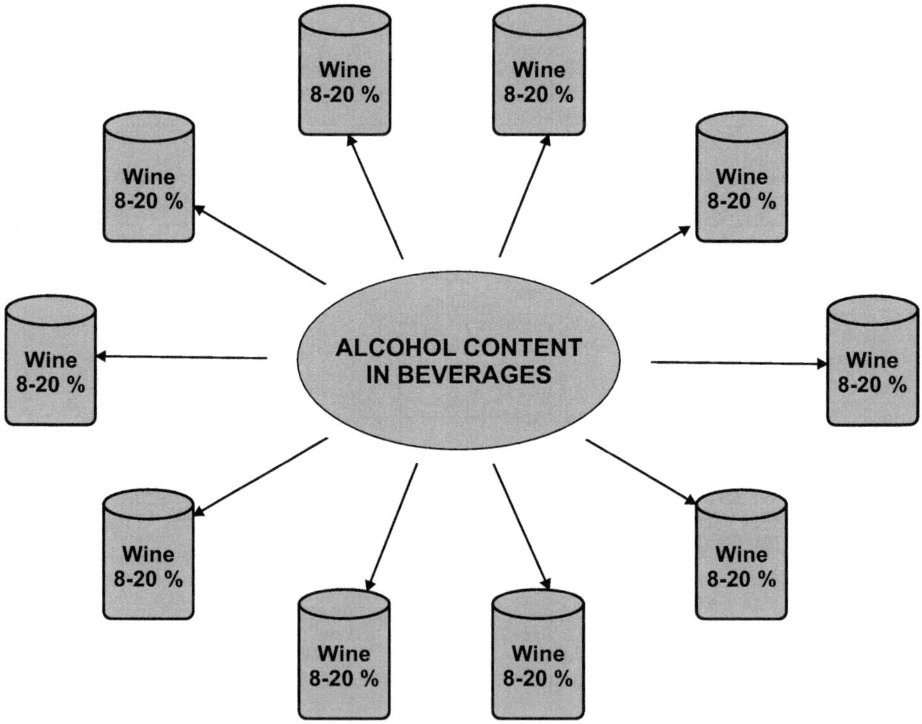

PREVENTING ALCOHOL ADDICTION:-

Prevention of alcohol addiction is a challenge, the person with an alcohol addiction need himself to contribute in the treatment with proper involvement. A rehabilitation process may be required if necessary for the treatment of the alcoholics. The three main lines of treatment along with rehabilitation are:-

Drug therapy, Counseling, Nutritional changes.
Alcohol treatment may involve several different treatment methods. It's important that alcoholics is willing to participate in recovery programme. This will help to heal the withdrawal symptoms.

Treatment of Alcoholism

Although often neglected, we need to give special attention to our young community who have never used alcohol.

The old saying **"Preventing addiction is more effective than curing it"** may seem idealistic, but it demonstrates a mindset that Indians need to adopt. While many programmes aim at presenting alternatives to addicts, we need to remember the community that has never been addicted or used alcohol extensively.

To help communities prevent alcohol abuse, some basic prevention ideas include:

- **Promotion of Health:** The community needs to promote healthy lifestyles through personal and cultural practices. By setting an example of health you will discourage damaging and dangerous lifestyles.
- **Focus on people and encouragement of social interaction:** Promotion of social interaction between old and young generations can only be done in a social environment. Create interactive environment through organized activities so that all ages can take part in it.
- **Local involvement of young people and respect for cultural value:** The activities you chose should focus on young people. Be sure to respect cultural traditions of the community.
- **Encouragement of positive alternatives:** Develop these alternatives with cultural values in mind, and understanding what appeals to the younger generation.
- **Long – term perspective:** Don't be discouraged if results aren't immediate. Preventing drug takes time – keeping a long term perspective is important.

- **Community development:** Focus on developing the fundamentals of your community, Education, Health and social services, Housing, Sanitation, and income generating activities are important ideas to focus on.

REFERENCE:

1. D. Daniel, D. Shetty, G.J. Jose, J. Haritha, J. Ravi, L. Pillai. Attitude of college students towards alcohol consumption in Manglore. *Nitte University journal of Health Science*. **2015**, 5(1), 37 – 39
2. N. Nakay. A study of the alcohol consumption patterns and their preference of liquor over wine amongst the youth in Manipal. *Journal of Biomedical and Health*. **2016**, 4(3), 58-62
3. P. Murthy. Culture and alcohol use in India. *World Cultural psychiatry research Review*. **2015**, 4(2), 27-39.

Editors' Note

Understanding fundamental concepts related to Alcohol use in diverse cultures give a reflection of probably of prevalent of alcoholism in that social setup. The general understanding of ill health effects of excessive use of alcohol can play preventive measure of alcohol use particularly in young generation.

❑❑❑

For Product Safety Concerns and Information please contact our EU representative GPSR@taylorandfrancis.com Taylor & Francis Verlag GmbH, Kaufingerstraße 24, 80331 München, Germany

Batch number: 10725798

Printed by Printforce, the Netherlands